Move
Yourself

Move Yourself

The Cooper Clinic Medical Director's
Guide to All the Healing
Benefits of Exercise
(Even a Little!)

TEDD MITCHELL, M.D.
TIM CHURCH, M.D., Ph. D.
MARTIN ZUCKER

WILEY

John Wiley & Sons, Inc.

Illustrations in chapters 10 and 11 by Bonita Versh (www.bonitaversh.com).

Published by John Wiley & Sons, Inc., Hoboken, New Jersey
Published simultaneously in Canada

For general information about our other products and services, please contact our Customer Care Department within the United States at (800) 762-2974, outside the United States at (317) 572-3993 or fax (317) 572-4002.

Wiley also publishes its books in a variety of electronic formats. Some content that appears in print may not be available in electronic books. For more information about Wiley products, visit our web site at www.wiley.com.

Library of Congress Cataloging-in-Publication Data:

Mitchell, Tedd, date.
  Move yourself : the Cooper Clinic medical director's guide to all the healing benefits of exercise (even a little!) / Tedd Mitchell, Tim Church, and Martin Zucker.
      p. cm.
  Includes bibliographical references and index.
  ISBN 978-0-470-04223-6 (cloth)
  1. Exercise—Health aspects. 2. Physical fitness. I. Church, Tim, 1965–
II. Zucker, Martin III. Title.
RA781.M587 2007
613.7—dc22   2008000279

Printed in the United States of America

10 9 8 7 6 5 4 3 2 1

To my father, Clayton Mitchell, M.D., for leading me to medicine;
to Kenneth Cooper, M.D., and Larry Gibbons, M.D., for
introducing me to the grand world of preventive medicine;
and to my wife, Janet Tornelli-Mitchell, M.D.,
and my children, Katherine, Charlie, and Chris,
for making my life a joy every day.

— *Tedd Mitchell*

To my parents, Lucy and Tom Church, and my brothers, Jeff and
Brian, for their continual support; to Natalie, my wife,
and to our children, Lucy Jean and Charlie, for giving me
meaning and purpose to this crazy adventure
called life; and to my Birmingham family for
their love and for helping me keep it real.

— *Tim Church*

To those mighty moms of Ottawa—Carole and Chantale—who
make physical activity part of their daily routine.

— *Martin Zucker*

CONTENTS

ACKNOWLEDGMENTS

To Steve Blair, P.E.D., for his profound impact on the science and public awareness of fitness, and for so much of the solid research that this book is based on.

To Janet Tornelli-Mitchell, M.D., for enlivening and enlarging the female perspectives in our book.

To Conrad Earnest, Ph.D., for his insights on nutritional supplements, and to Jay Ashmore, Ph.D., for his input on weight loss.

To Georgia Kostas, M.P.H., R.D., the former director of nutrition at the Cooper Clinic, for sharing her twenty-five years' experience in the nutrition field. Her unique perspective will help our readers effectively and nutritionally reduce calories as part of a physical activity and diet program for waist removal and weight loss.

To Kathy Duran-Thal, R.D., the clinic's present director, for sharing a commonsense approach to eating for health.

To Erin Sinclair, Jason Wallace, and especially Claire Avant, for valuable feedback and helping locate once sedentary but now active interviewees.

To Balkis Wiggins, Isabel Arista, and Christina Turbeville for their inspirational stories of transformation.

To the magic pen of Bonita Versh, artist and animator extraordinaire, for her wonderful line renditions of strength and stretching exercises.

To Mariann Madsen, for being such a reliable and cheerful emissary between busy authors.

To Bernard C. K. Choi, Ph.D., of Canada's Centre for Chronic Disease Prevention and Control, for sharing the important perspectives he and other leading public health officials have developed about "diseases of comfort."

PART ONE

The Power
of Movement

1

A Little Activity Goes a Long Way

Sedentary: From the Latin word *sedentarius*, meaning "sitting, remaining in one place." Pertaining to animals who move about little or who, like a barnacle, are permanently attached to something.

Everybody has excuses for not exercising, and Tina was no exception, although, as a hospital food and nutrition director, she should have known better. It was her job to teach people how to eat better and live healthier.

Nevertheless, she had let herself go. She had a membership at a gym, and a treadmill and two stationary bikes at home. But while she was working and raising four kids, the struggles and challenges of life overcame her good intentions.

"I got tired just thinking of going to the gym after a busy eight- or ten-hour day, working out for forty minutes, and then coming home to cook dinner. And so from about age forty-five to sixty, I didn't take good care of myself," she said. "Instead of using the treadmill, I would hang my clothes on it. Instead of following the diet I preached to others, I ate much more rich food than I should have. And, I have to confess, as my kids got older and I didn't have to jump up and down during meals to get this and that for them, I enjoyed what I was eating more than ever."

As others often do when they reach a milestone in life, Tina did a reality check at age sixty and realized that her energy had been sputtering for about five years. Her weight had ballooned from 135 to 170 pounds.

3

She had chronic lower back pain and a touch of arthritis in her knees for which she took pain medication on and off.

For her sixtieth birthday, her children gave her a party and took lots of pictures. When she saw herself in the photos, Tina was appalled.

"You are fat, lady," she said to herself. "You are gross. You go around telling diabetic and cardiac patients what to do, but look at you. You don't practice what you preach."

Tina said the pictures jump-started her quest to improve her health. She began looking for a program that could help her reach her goal and found one that inspired her: a program that teaches adults how to convert daily routines into exercise.

"I took to the concept immediately," Tina said. "There was no gym. No sweating. No need for a workout."

She started off with something utterly simple and nonchallenging: the 2-minute walk.

"I'd be sitting at my desk for a while and realize I needed to get up and do something," she said. "So I would get up and walk for two minutes in the hallways. I did that ten times a day. That's twenty minutes. Later I might do five minutes five times a day, or ten minutes three times a day. It all depended on my day. But that's how I got back into better condition. That's how physical activity became doable for me."

Tina said she soon started considering every activity in her day a potential source of exercise.

"Vacuuming the house became a ten-minute exercise, and fifteen if I did the steps in the house as well. Walking the stairs at the hospital instead of taking the elevator became a routine. And parking my car as far away from my destination as was practical.

"I'm a TV addict. But now instead of watching commercials I walk the commercials. I can walk around the house seventeen times at a moderate speed during a typical commercial break. If the weather is good, I go out the front door, walk around the house, and come in the back door, or walk to the end of the driveway and back several times. Who needs all those commercials?

"Often my husband joins me, or one of the grandkids, so it becomes fun. And when I go to any of the grandkids' soccer or baseball games, I'll walk around the field instead of sitting there the whole time."

After about four months, Tina lost 10 pounds and noticed that her energy level was back to where it had been when she was much younger.

"At the level before the kids wore me out," she joked. After six months, she realized she wasn't hurting anymore, that she had no need for pain medication.

"Before, my kids were worried about my health, and now they see the changes and cheer me on."

Tina reversed the direction of her health by stepping forward—literally and figuratively. She sat less and moved more. It was nothing dramatic but it was enough to remove herself from the ranks of the sedentary, unhealthy, and habitually tired majority of Americans (and most other Westerners as well). She went from being busy and inactive to being busy and active.

The program that recharged Tina's life was influenced by ideas and research generated at the Cooper Aerobics Center in Dallas, Texas, the leading medical fitness facility in the world. Two of us have been intimately involved in this amazing operation—Dr. Mitchell as medical director of the center's renowned clinic and Dr. Church as the medical director of its research branch.

Since 1970 more than eighty-five thousand patients and many thousands of fitness study participants have come through our doors. We record the details of their health, diet, activity, and cause of death when they die. This ongoing collection of information constitutes the world's largest fitness database, funded since 1984 by the National Institute of Aging. Our own research specialists, as well as researchers from all over the world, tap into this huge bank of data to study and report on the relationship between physical activity and health, disease risk factors, and causes of death.

In both our clinical and research activities, we see many sedentary individuals. For instance, about a third of our patients are employees sent by their companies for checkups. They come because their companies pay their way. Many of them have typically unhealthy lifestyle habits and truly represent the sedentary state of America.

The large number and variety of individuals we see give us unequaled clarity on the impact that physical activity has on health. We know unequivocally, beyond any shadow of a doubt, that a sedentary lifestyle directly *causes* chronic disease and a shorter life span regardless of whether you are thin, overweight, or obese. Yet this simple fact of life is commonly ignored, overlooked, or underestimated, even by doctors.

The direct and indirect costs of idleness in the United States alone exceed $150 billion a year, or roughly 15 percent of the country's health-care budget. Twice as many people die from sedentary living than from viruses and bacteria, and more die from inactivity than from firearms, illicit use of drugs, sexually transmitted diseases, and automobile accidents combined. In a 2002 analysis of medical expenditures among state health plan members, researchers from Blue Cross Blue Shield of Minnesota linked physical inactivity to 31 percent of heart disease and stroke cases, incidents of colon cancer and osteoporosis, and nearly 12 percent of anxiety and depression cases.

According to government statistics, approximately 75 percent of U.S. adults are sedentary. By definition that means they sit most of the time and are physically active for fewer than the recommended 150 minutes per week. The percentage is really misleading because official statistics rely on self-reporting surveys where individuals estimate their own activity level. When you ask people to fill out questionnaires, they grossly overestimate the time they spend exercising. So data indicating that just a quarter of Americans meet the general criteria for physical activity probably are an exaggeration.

Frank Booth, Ph.D., a professor of physiology at the University of Missouri, has coined the term *sedentary death syndrome* to describe the impact of the ongoing physical decline of the human species. "A subpopulation of genes, which have functioned to support physical activity for survival through most of humankind's existence, require daily exercise to maintain long-term health and vitality," Booth points out. "Type 2 diabetes is an example of a sedentary death syndrome condition, as it is almost entirely preventable with physical activity."

The tragedy in all of this is that most sedentary people can easily convert their self-destructive "deathstyle" into a healthy lifestyle. We know because we have seen it happen repeatedly. What's more, it can be accomplished with just minutes a day of low-dose physical activity. That's enough to reap a high dose of benefits—starting within days.

If the notion of rigorous exercise turns you off, this book has some very enticing, comforting, and practical information for you. To make yourself healthier—as Tina did—you don't have to go out and jog or run a marathon. You don't have to join a gym.

Our research has also given us a unique perspective on the overweight and obesity problem that experts say makes people more vulnerable to illness and early death. The experts predict, in fact, that excess weight will soon pass smoking as the number-one preventable cause of premature death. Our research sees the weight issue differently. We say that the problem is not so much the weight, but the lack of physical activity. Regular activity, even if you are obese, protects your health more than if you are thin but physically inactive. Whether you are underweight, normal weight, or overweight—a lack of routine physical activity puts you at higher risk of developing premature disease.

To us, a sedentary lifestyle already represents the overall number-one preventable cause of premature death. Becoming physically active—even to just a minimal degree—is probably as important to our health as quitting smoking is for a smoker.

How Much Activity Do You Need to Be Healthy?

In 1970 Kenneth Cooper, M.D., founded our center after he wrote the best seller *Aerobics*, the book that started the jogging craze. *Aerobics* changed the way people, including medical professionals, regarded physical fitness. Until its publication, relatively few devotees took regular exercise seriously. Most people regarded time spent on physical activity as a luxury, certainly not as a necessity.

In the following years, Dr. Cooper championed the idea that the more you exercised, the better your health would be. If you walked, you should walk faster and farther. If you walked fast, you should jog. If you jogged, you should jog faster and farther. Push it. Do more. That was the mantra of fitness—then.

It was our own database that changed this perspective. Beginning in 1989, we began to see evidence that even a little physical activity goes a long way. The evidence has grown ever since. We've learned that the benefits of fitness are assuredly not limited to high-performance athletes, gym addicts, or those who "grind it out." As our most recent studies indicate, the benefits start with much less activity than is commonly recommended.

In the 1990s we learned through a study appropriately dubbed "Project Active" that you can readily accumulate activity minutes throughout

**PHYSICAL ACTIVITY
VS. EXERCISE**

Physical activity means movement. It comprises simple things you can do in your daily life to get you moving and off the chair or couch, or away from the TV or computer.

Exercise is a type of physical activity for which you set time aside for bodily exertion. You can be very physically active yet never actually exercise.

the day, even on workdays, to get health benefits similar to those gained by somebody who works out at a fitness center. You can lower your blood pressure, lose body fat, protect your heart, and have a lot of fun in the process just by logging 30 activity minutes as part of your regular daily schedule. During this time we began recommending the step counter, a simple device you can clip onto your clothes. Keeping count of your steps enables you to challenge yourself each day to take more steps than you did the day before. It is also a fun way to explore myriad innovative ways to accumulate activity minutes. Over the years the step counter has proven to be a winner, a great motivator for starting or restarting even the most sedentary folks on a fitness quest. Later in the book we will show you how to use it.

Our Postmenopausal Study:
Less *Is* Good

No single piece of research illustrates the promise of low-dose physical activity on fitness and health better than a recent study we did with postmenopausal women. More than one in three American women are postmenopausal. When they enter this stage of life, their risk of heart attack or stroke increases dramatically.

We don't have a lot of good therapies to reduce the risk for heart attack or stroke. Hormone replacement has been disappointing, and many doctors now oppose it.

We wanted to find out whether physical activity could lower the risk of such incidents. We know that fitness declines as a person ages. Experts believe, as the chart below dramatically shows, that the rate of fitness decline is about 1 to 2 percent a year. We also know that one of the strongest predictors of premature death is a low level of fitness. So to us,

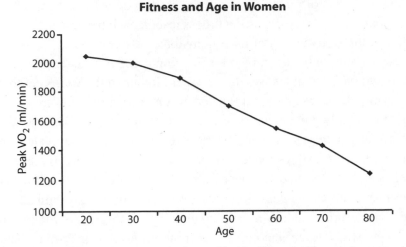

The decline of fitness in women as determined by VO$_2$ max (the maximum amount of oxygen the body can consume during intense exercise), a measurement used to determine an individual's aerobic fitness. (Source: Fleg JL, Morrell CH, Bos AG, et al. *Circulation*, 2005.)

fitness represents a natural variable to improve in an effort to impact longevity.

In 2005 we designed a study to determine how much regular physical activity postmenopausal women would require to either maintain fitness—that is, to prevent a fitness decline—or to increase fitness in order to improve the premature death rate and overall quality of life. We enrolled 464 women with an average age of fifty-seven into the six-month study. It was the largest single physical activity experiment conducted with postmenopausal women in the world and probably the largest conducted with women at a single site.

We recruited participants by advertising in the Dallas-area media. On average the respondents were more than 30 pounds overweight, had elevated blood pressure, and were extremely sedentary. Many were beginning to have substantial health issues. We felt our participants were fairly representative of a large segment of American women.

The women came to our center and alternated between walking on a treadmill and riding a stationary bicycle. The intensity level was very low, barely enough to cause a sweat—a walking pace just above a stroll and a cycling pace slightly exceeding light pedaling. We looked at three different durations of physical activity: approximately 75, 150, and 225 minutes per week. We performed a fitness test on each participant before the start of the study and after its conclusion.

Doctors commonly recommend 150 minutes of physical activity a week, based on 30 minutes five days a week. In our study, we found that even 75 minutes a week—accumulated in three or four sessions—was enough to not only prevent a loss of fitness over the course of six months but to actually increase a woman's fitness level. That's the equivalent of about 15 minutes five days a week. To be sure, the benefits of 150 minutes a week were greater, and the benefits of 225 minutes were somewhat greater than that, but the gains from minimum activity were significant.

We were surprised and even amazed at how well the 75-minute group fared in the study. Even one-half the common prescription for physical activity paid off substantially in terms of health benefits and the potential to neutralize vulnerability for many diseases.

The results were eye-opening:

- All groups involved in the study lost two pounds on average. (This included the control group, which did not participate in any physical activities. We think that hearing us speak about eating healthier inspired them to make dietary changes at home, which in turn caused their weight loss.)

- Only the physical activity groups lost dangerous belly fat. (You will learn more about this type of fat in the next chapter.) The participants were delighted to see their waist circumference shrink by 1 to 2 inches on average.

- We saw improvement in blood sugar in all activity groups.

- Among physical activity participants there was an across-the-board improvement in heart-rate variability, which would reduce a tendency toward dangerous heart rhythms.

- Out of all the study's participants, 91 percent completed the entire study and 97 percent complied fully with what we asked of them. We regard this high participation rate as both a reflection of the good work of our staff as well as the reality that a simple physical activity program is very doable even for sedentary women. Our participants were not overwhelmed. Those who dropped out usually did so because of a major life event, such as illness in the family.

Afterward, many of the participants told us the experience was a blessing at a time of life when they otherwise would have kept going downhill physically. They continued to stay active, to enjoy their new-found energy, and to get more out of life. Some mentioned that their clothes fit better. One woman said she got her curves back. Another said the study changed her life. Her family and friends kept telling her how good she looked, and her self-image soared.

Our study offers an affirmative and practical answer to the frequently asked question among fitness researchers: Do sedentary individuals achieve an improved fitness level if they perform less physical activity than the commonly recommended amount? Our study says yes, significantly so, and even at a time in life when their fitness level has dropped considerably.

We try to steer people in the direction of 30 minutes on most and preferably all days of the week, but the study's striking result is that even 15 minutes a day of low-intensity activity has big benefits. That has big practical implications. Among aging or very unfit populations, 150 minutes of activity each week may not be realistic. However, at least 75 minutes should be doable and will help deter fitness decline and reduce the risk of dying prematurely. A more modest goal, yet with solid gains, may keep you on a fitness program.

At our clinic, sedentary patients regularly tell staff doctors that they feel better even if they can only manage walking two or three times a week for 15 minutes at a time or riding a stationary bike for as little as 5 minutes three times a day. That's only 45 minutes a week! It proves to us that any level of activity is better than none. A little bit seems to go a long way. For us, and indeed for public health policy, that's big news and a big payoff. And that's why we wrote this book.

Why Physical Activity Works So Well and So Fast

Physical activity affects every cell in the body, which is precisely why it is such good mind-body medicine and why you pay a heavy price for being sedentary.

Most people know that physical activity is a good thing. They just don't know how good. They seem to equate physical activity with leaving the mayonnaise off their sandwich at lunchtime. In other words, it is not such a big deal whether you do it. How wrong they are! Briefly, here's what physical activity does for you:

Movement increases your blood flow.   Nothing ensures good blood flow and prompt delivery of raw materials to the trillions of cells in your body as well as physical activity does. The cells depend on the oxygen and nutrients supplied by the blood to do their various jobs—from the heart muscle cells that keep your heart pumping to the brain cells that keep you thinking and coordinating your countless activities.

If your gas line gets clogged, your car sputters. If your blood vessels are clogged and the blood delivery is sluggish, your cells can't do their jobs well. You sputter. In time you'll develop sickness wherever cells are the most compromised. Healthy cells make up healthy organs and healthy organs make up healthy bodies, so good blood flow is critical.

Movement makes your nervous system work better.   Nerve cells also benefit from better blood flow. Physical activity is able to quickly shift the 100 billion neurons in your brain from a revved, stressed state—more vulnerable to dangerous cardiac rhythms and heart attacks—to a relaxed state.

We routinely measure the electrical impulses in the heart and find that physical activity rapidly changes the level of heart nervousness. That's important because the cardiac electrical system controls the speed of your heartbeat. You want this system working smoothly so that it efficiently responds to changing demands for oxygen, speeding up the rate when you are active and slowing it down when you are at rest.

Movement improves your metabolism. Metabolism refers to the ongoing chemical processes within living cells and organisms that are necessary for the maintenance of life. For example, muscle tissue is the biggest single consumer of glucose (blood sugar that has been broken down from dietary carbohydrates) and a minimal amount of physical activity helps keep muscles happily utilizing blood sugar. This helps prevent blood sugar and insulin levels from rising dangerously in the body—a condition that leads to diabetes and damage to nerves, blood vessels, and the liver. Physical activity also helps the body clear excess fats (triglyc-erides) from the bloodstream, preventing them from being deposited in the liver or spleen, or near the heart.

No pill or substance can produce as many health dividends as physi-cal activity can. When you add up activity's basic contributions to your well-being the sum total is astounding. Here's a short list of the benefits:

- Better utilization of blood sugar (meaning better protection against diabetes)
- Reduced blood pressure
- Lower risk of cardiovascular disease (heart attacks and stroke)
- Lower risk of certain cancers, such as colon cancer
- Lower risk of metabolic syndrome (a symptomless condition that sets up the body for serious chronic diseases)
- Reduced stress
- Improved mood, reducing incidents of depression
- Improved bone and joint health
- Improved recovery from illness by promoting the body's healing mechanisms
- Healthier and stronger muscles—a key to healthy aging
- Positive weight redistribution in your body—you look better and your clothes fit better
- Less belly fat that is dangerous to your health

Quality of Life—
the Best Motivator

Did you know that even if you have been inactive for years, you begin to derive benefits the moment you launch into physical activity? Within days of starting our program, formerly sedentary people often tell us how much better they feel and how much more energy they have. It can work that fast. It's as if their bodies are saying thank you for giving them what they need. If you are feeling down, for instance, just go out and take a walk, and when you come back you'll likely be feeling better.

This kind of patient feedback about improved quality of life is what really seems to get people to stick with physical activity after they have started on a program. The statistics bear that out. For this book we crunched numbers on more than ten thousand patients—both men and women, sedentary and active—who have gone through our clinic since 1998. Among them were 1,077 individuals in the low-fitness category, 3,555 who were moderately fit, and 5,679 who were highly fit.

We analyzed specific quality-of-life responses, which they had given to simple yes or no questions on medical history forms: questions asking, for example, whether they had frequent heartburn or lower back pain. The survey produced compelling evidence for the big difference physical activity makes on everyday living, not just on medical test scores. Here are some examples of positive results gained from an activity program:

- Improved sex drive and reduced impotence
- Improved energy, both short- and long-term
- Improved sleep
- Reduced snoring
- Less heartburn
- Reduced need to urinate at night
- Reduced joint, muscle, and back pain
- Fewer headaches
- Improved memory in older people

Do you know of any pill or substance that can produce all these quality-of-life dividends? These improvements, of which even most doctors are unaware, are fabulous motivators for sustaining physical activity. Nothing makes us happier as physicians than when previously inactive and unhealthy patients tell us they started a physical activity routine, stayed with it, and now feel great. Some of these are patients we have hounded for years, nagging them at every checkup about the dangers of inactivity.

So why, we ask, are they sticking with it now after all these years? They'll often answer:

- "My back isn't bothering me for the first time in years."
- "I sleep better."
- "I'm not snoring anymore."
- "I don't have heartburn anymore."
- "You said that I would need to take more medication if I didn't do something about my [blood sugar, blood pressure, etc.], so I decided to do something."

Something clicked along life's journey for these patients. Maybe they just got tired of our badgering them. Or maybe they went through a health crisis. Whatever got them started, it's often the realization that they feel a whole lot better that keeps them active for the long term. Of course, improved blood and medical tests usually give objective backing to subjective improvements, but in our experience that's not what gets people to stick with it. It's the quality-of-life and daily existence factors that do it—factors that medical professionals tend to dismiss but which we find are real motivators. Simply said, we see happier and healthier patients when they stick to an activity program.

We do not for a moment discount other pillars of a healthy lifestyle, such as nutrition and stress reduction. They are extremely important, and in fact, we cover these elements in all patient education programs at our center.

What's Your Activity Level?

We've got two simple ways for you to determine just how sedentary you are. First, answer the simple self-assessment questions below about your activity level. Second, determine your actual daily activity with a step counter.

Based on our experience with thousands of subjects in our research projects, we know people tend to distort their survey answers to appear more active than they really are. For that reason, we put more emphasis on the second part of this test—the step counter.

Answer yes or no to the following questions:

Do you have a job where you spend most of the day at a desk?

When you get home from school or work, do you eat supper in front of the TV?

Do you reserve your evenings for TV or a movie?

Do your weekend plans usually consist largely of sedentary activities, such as eating, drinking, and sitting around?

Are you unlikely to get 20 or 30 minutes of physical activity a day on most days of the week?

Do you pay somebody to do your housework or yard work?

When you walk into a two- or three-story building, do you take the elevator to go to a higher floor?

If you have a dog, does someone in your family other than you routinely walk it?

Does walking a block or going up a flight of stairs make you out of breath?

Do you own exercise equipment that gets more use as a clothes hanger or laundry rack than as it is intended to be used?

If you answered yes to seven or more questions, you are super-sedentary. You should change your ways. If you answered yes to four to six questions, you are in the sedentary ballpark and could improve your fitness level. Four or more yes answers make you a candidate for our Plan A startup program, which you will find in part two of this book.

If you answered yes to three questions or fewer, you are doing pretty well. Check out our Plan B recommendations in part two of this book.

For the real test of your physical activity, we would like you to buy an inexpensive step counter and see how many steps you take in an average day. This exercise will confirm your activity level. You can pick up a step counter (sometimes called a "pedometer") at any sporting goods store or order one from our center (on the Internet at www.coopercomplete.com/books.php/, or by phone toll-free at 1-888-393-2221). A step counter is a great tool for determining how active you are—or aren't—and also to jump-start you into a physical activity program.

You can clip a step counter to your pants or skirt (for more information on the step counter, refer to chapter 5). Put it on in the morning and take it off at night before bedtime. Make a note of how many steps you take each day for a two- or three-day period. Don't do anything different. Just follow your usual routine.

No one knows exactly how many steps an average American takes each day, but from our research and from patients' responses, we figure that an average sedentary person takes fewer than five thousand steps a day. So if you fall below that number, you are distinctly sedentary. Figure it this way:

Below 4,500 steps means you're very sedentary.

4,500–5,500 steps: You're sedentary.

5,500–7,500 steps: Keep it up. You're headed in the right direction.

7,500–8,500: You're active. But it wouldn't hurt to add even more steps.

8,500 and above: You're good and active. Stick with it.

After doing the test, hang on to your step counter. You're going to rely on it to move yourself out of the sedentary category and into the active one. You'll be amazed, as you will find out in chapter 5, how much fun the step counter can make this process.

How to Use This Book

Our book is loaded with lessons we have learned from thousands of patients and study participants. Think of it as a road map to transport you directly to your fitness, health, and weight goals. There's something here for everybody.

In part one you'll find information that you need to know about physical activity:

- A strong argument about why physical activity trumps weight loss—being skinnier does not necessarily make you healthier.

- The lowdown on killer belly fat and how easy it is to neutralize it.

- A clear understanding of how physical activity protects you against a wide range of common ailments such as diabetes, heart attacks, and the insidious metabolic syndrome.

- Never before published information from our patient survey revealing how physical activity improves core quality-of-life issues related to mood, energy, sleep, digestion, elimination, and sex drive.

In part two you'll get the practical, how-to information:

- For people who are currently sedentary, we have laid out a practical and enjoyable prescription for infusing daily life with low-dose physical activity. We call it "Plan A for Active." It can restore zest and vitality to even the most sluggish of persons within thirty days. We'll show you how to start up gently and safely, and how to stick with it; and we'll give you effective strategies for overcoming the usual reasons that people slack off. We've also included recommendations on how to incorporate some better eating choices—not a diet—after you have sustained Plan A for a month. Some easy-to-make food upgrades multiply your benefits. You get healthier bit by bit, step by step, bite by bite.

- For people who graduate from Plan A, or who are already active and want to maximize their functional fitness, we have compiled a comprehensive approach to physical activity. We call this "Plan B for Balance." Here is where we use the term *exercise*, and have you set aside time specifically for physical activity to boost the heart, lungs, and muscles, and to increase joint flexibility for better mobility. We recommend basic fitness principles relating to frequency, intensity, and time of exercise. You apply these principles as you pursue cardiovascular, strength, and stretching fitness in a balanced way, and focus on more than just one single aspect of exercising.

- For individuals with excess abdominal fat and weight, we have put together a weight-loss program—"Plan C for Calories." We'll show you how to burn more and eat less, with a program that includes a more intense exercise schedule and a restricted-calorie diet. Long ago we learned that those two things are necessary in order to lose weight and *keep it off*.

2

Focus on Fitness, Not Thinness

It's not what you weigh but where you weigh.

—Anonymous

W e Westerners are a fat-phobic lot. We live by the bathroom scale, our self-image riding on every rise or fall of the pointer. For most, the pointer is also an indicator of health status. In the pages ahead we hope to emancipate you from such misguided thinking.

When patients discuss their health with us, the first words out of their mouths usually are about their weight. "I put on five pounds since the last time I was here, and so I'm really in bad shape, and I think my health is suffering as a result."

There's nothing surprising in such responses, since our society is obsessed with thinness. Most of us believe that weight is virtually synonymous with health, and we have been bombarded until numb with warnings about the obesity epidemic and its devastating health ramifications.

Weight, weight loss, and diets sell books and magazine articles, and if you are a diet expert, you get on the top TV shows. People want to talk about weight. We spend $30 billion a year on weight-loss programs and products. Still, we get heavier and heavier. We keep investing in a losing strategy and focusing on the wrong target. Many experts have begun questioning the science behind all the obesity claims and wondering whether it's science or profit that is driving the weight-loss mania.

Most studies investigating the connection between weight and health fail to give adequate emphasis to physical activity. Researchers usually rely on simple self-report questionnaires in which exaggerating the amount of personal physical activity tends to increase proportionally with the respondents' weight. When calculating health risks, physical activity means as much in the consideration of obesity as tobacco use does for lung cancer.

We believe physical inactivity is a paramount cause of our rampant weight problem. To us, getting yourself physically active is the first step to health and weight loss. Yet physical activity consistently fails to get equal billing with diet-focused weight loss or anything near the attention it deserves.

Beginning in 1999 we first reported that physically active overweight people—even those who are obese—are much healthier than their skinnier but sedentary peers. In a study we published that year, in collaboration with health and longevity expert Ralph Paffenbarger of Stanford University, we found that a low fitness level was a strong and independent predictor of cardiovascular disease and premature death from all causes. The fitness factor was as significant as diabetes and other cardiovascular risks, and was relevant even when people were underweight or obese.

Our study looked at the medical records of more than twenty-five thousand men who had undergone examinations at our center from 1970 to 1993. The average follow-up period after the initial examination was ten years. As the graph on the next page shows, fit men with a body mass index categorizing them as obese had virtually the same risk of dying during the follow-up period as the so-called normal-weight men. Unfit obese men had three times the risk of dying.

Our big database and the outcomes with our individual patients have repeatedly demonstrated that people moderately or highly fit—even if overweight or obese—have a much lower risk of dying prematurely compared to individuals of low fitness. Keep in mind it takes only 150 minutes a week—or even less, as we have seen—of physical activity to keep out of the unfit category.

Obviously, there is a point where weight does have an impact on health. The fitness-health connection starts to unravel when you move up into higher levels of obesity. You can't be hundreds of pounds overweight and be healthy. We aren't talking about such people here, although we have had some in our center and have helped them regain their health with a comprehensive program that included routine physical activity.

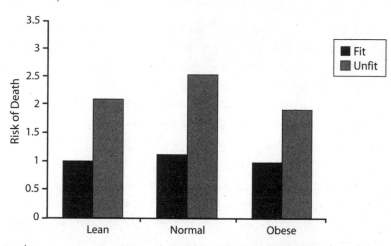

Fit-Fat and Mortality in Men

This graph represents our 1999 analysis of how fitness affects the risk of dying. More than 25,000 male patients were monitored. The body mass index group on the left represents lean patients, with normal weight patients in the center, and on the right, obese patients. The graph provides a striking comparison—and argument—for the benefits of fitness at any weight. (Source: Wei M, Kampert JB, Barlow CE, et al. *JAMA*, 1999.)

The Thinness Obsession

We strongly believe that fitness is more important than the elusive concept of normal weight. What is normal, anyway? It's a figure developed by the insurance industry to identify higher- and lower-risk individuals. For many people, getting down to an arbitrary weight level borders on the impossible. Some individuals have body types that are naturally heavier. So a lower "norm" may not be reachable or sustainable or necessary for good health. Why set yourself up for defeat? If you constantly and unsuccessfully wage war to lose some extra pounds and keep them off, you are wasting your time. Forget the weight. Instead, get fit, even if just moderately.

We give many talks to lay audiences. Many worried people in the audience have told us that their doctors have recommended they lose 10, 15, 20, or more pounds—goals that for them are difficult or impossible to achieve. These recommendations are frequently given without taking eating or physical activity habits into consideration. People comment that they feel great and are doing all the right things. They are physically active and eat right, but for the life of them they cannot lose the weight. The failure worries them.

Our response is simple: Don't focus on your weight so much. You may be where you belong. Focus on your behavior—diet and activity— not the pounds. Genetically, not everyone can be skinny. Everyone, however, can be healthier and more fit.

Behavior is a much better measure of your present and future health than any scale, and being heavy in a nonextreme sense is not necessarily unhealthy, as long as you stay active and eat right.

Usually there's a ripple of relief in the audience. We've defused a common concern. The notion of being unhealthy because of a few pounds is an infuriating and stressful myth for someone who is regularly active. Unfortunately, the myth thrives far and wide and drives people to undertake unnecessary and futile dieting.

Stop Worrying about Your Weight

Janet Tornelli-Mitchell, M.D., coauthor Tedd Mitchell's wife, is a staff physician at our clinic. She sees many women for checkups and treatment who are weight worriers to the extreme. She tries to help them refocus their priorities.

"I tell them to stop buying the magazines with the girls on the cover who are far too thin, who have had cosmetic surgery, or whose images have been enhanced by computer graphic technology. You can't compare yourself with those images. You can't really hope to look like that. Identifying with those pictures will only make you frustrated and even depressed.

"What you need to be is healthy, even if that means that you have ten or more extra pounds that you haven't been able to shed since you had your children. If you are physically active and trying to eat healthy, that's a whole lot better than being five-foot-eight and ninety pounds and smoking cigarettes to keep your weight down.

"You don't have to be skinny. You have to be healthy. You can have extra pounds and still be healthier than a skinny person."

To illustrate her point, Dr. Tornelli-Mitchell often shares this personal story with her patients:

"Years ago after having my children I had gained ten pounds and was having a hard time losing the extra weight. One day a friend came over and suggested we take a walk. She was one of those people who took great pride in her thinness. She wore a size two dress and never hesitated to remind others of that fact. Yet she was terribly out of shape. We set out to do a mile and after just a short distance I thought she was going to collapse. She became red-faced and short of breath. I got scared. Here I was, packing more than ten pounds I didn't really want, but not terribly concerned. I remember thinking at the time about how much better off I was, being a bit heavier but fit, than somebody who was a size two and unfit. Over time, the extra weight came off, but the incident made an indelible impression in my mind regarding the importance of fitness over thinness."

If you are a woman reading this book, you need to know that you can be a size two and be a physical disaster. Or you can be like Dr. Tornelli-Mitchell, more concerned about her health than her dress size, who can go out and walk a couple of miles without a problem. The choice is obvious.

Dr. Tornelli-Mitchell says that some of her patients have very unrealistic ideas of what their weight should be. Here's a typical conversation she has with patients:

"What do you think your weight should be?"

"Oh, what I weighed in high school."

"I've got news for you. You'll probably never, ever weigh that again. So forget about it. As long as you have unrealistic goals, you are just going to set yourself up to fail. Instead, just think about getting physically active and losing a few pounds over the next year, something more realistic."

"But don't you think I need to lose more?"

"Lose a few pounds and then come back and we'll talk some more. I'm sure you'll be feeling a whole lot better when you return."

"I can do that."

Dr. Tornelli-Mitchell says her patients are hugely relieved.

We see the same relief with our male patients. As with all our patients, we ask what they think their ideal weight should be. One patient who weighed 247 pounds said he believed he should be 180.

"Why 180?" he was asked.

"That's what I weighed in high school."

"You don't have to weigh 180. You just need to be healthy."

When he was told that, and told why and how, his eyes lit up.

"I would like you, though, to get down to 220 pounds or so over time. You don't have to be in a rush. But I do need you to get active because that will make you healthier and protect you more than losing the weight, and in the process you will lose some weight. But don't make the weight your priority. Make the activity, and your health, your priority."

"I can sure do that."

The concern of patients over their "excess" pounds practically comes tumbling off their shoulders when they learn they don't need to maintain their high school weight in adulthood. The relief is immense.

Body Mass Index (BMI)

You've probably heard of the famous body mass index (BMI), a mathematical formula created to calculate a global standard for categorizing weight as underweight, normal, overweight, or obese. The BMI measurement is the ratio of the weight of the body in kilograms to the square of its height in meters.

While it's useful for looking at weight issues in the general population, the index is much less helpful when it comes to counseling individuals. What you weigh is not nearly as important as what your weight is composed of and where your weight is. Take two men, for instance, both 6 feet 2 inches tall and weighing 240 pounds. Using the BMI, both would be classified as obese (and therefore at risk for health problems).

Here's the problem. One of the men may be a sedentary businessman with a physique like Baby Huey, the bulbous-bellied duckling of comic and cartoon fame, while the other may be an extraordinarily athletic businessman with a physique like Arnold Schwarzenegger. Same height, same weight, but with vastly different body compositions—and hence with vastly different health risks.

The BMI also tends to be less accurate for older people, who put on more fat and lose muscle and bone with age. Nor does it take into account dangerous visceral fat, which we'll discuss in a moment.

Our experience at the Cooper Aerobics Center clearly indicates that fitness provides considerable protection for people of class I obesity

CALCULATE YOUR BODY MASS INDEX

If you are interested in knowing your individual BMI, the Centers for Disease Control and Prevention offers a BMI calculator at www.cdc.gov/nccdphp/dnpa/bmi/adult_BMI/english_bmi_calculator/bmi_calculator.htm. Just enter your height and weight, and click on the calculate button.

If you don't mind doing a bit of math, you can also easily calculate your BMI using the following simple formula:

Figure your height in inches (e.g., 63 inches).

Figure your height squared. Multiply your height in inches by itself (e.g., 63 x 63 = 3,969).

Divide your weight in pounds by your height squared (e.g, 120 pounds divided by 3,969). Then multiply by 703. The BMI total for someone 63 inches tall and weighing 120 pounds is 21.3, a "normal" rating.

The standard weight status categories associated with BMI ranges for adults are shown in the following table.

BMI	Weight Status
Below 18.5	Underweight
18.5–24.9	Normal
25.0–29.9	Overweight
30.0 and above	Obese

(BMI 30–34.9), and probably for those up to a 37 or 38 level in class II (BMI 35–39.9) as well.

Taking the Killer out of Killer Fat

To get to know your fat, take this quick quiz.

1. Where on your body does fat bother you the most?

   A. When it hangs from your arms

   B. When it pads your hips and thighs

   C. When it bulges out from your rear

   D. When it protrudes from your midsection

There's no right answer here. Different folks have different answers depending on their own self-image.

2. Which of these fat zones is the most hazardous to your health?

A. Arms

B. Hips and thighs

C. Butt

D. Midsection

For that there is one correct answer: D.

In addition to moving you off your chair and getting you more active, we hope this book will raise your awareness about body fat, particularly about what we call visceral adiposity (a fancy word for belly fat). A bulging middle means trouble—too much subcutaneous and visceral fat. There are two kinds of belly fat, depending on where the fat is stored. One is subcutaneous; that is, just beneath the skin—the fat you can pinch and try to diet away before bathing suit season arrives. From a health and medical standpoint, we are not really as concerned with it. It's the deeper, visceral fat that worries us the most, the padding that surrounds the liver and other abdominal organs. The more of it you have, the more at risk your health is.

Researchers started becoming aware of visceral fat in the 1980s, but only in recent years have they learned that this particular fat, distinct from other fat tissue in the body, appears to be particularly harmful. This inner padding acts like a factory zone, producing a steady stream of unhealthy substances that spill into the body. They include interleukin-6 and tumor necrosis factor, proteins that kindle a dangerous, low-level, chronic inflammation throughout the system. This type of constant inflammation underlies arterial disease. Indeed, individuals with excess fatty tissue tend to develop a prothrombotic state, meaning they are more prone to form plaque and blood vessel blockages, which in turn increase the danger of a heart attack. They also develop problems with blood sugar and an increased risk of diabetes.

Moreover, visceral fat secretions travel an expressway—the portal vein—straight to the liver and thus directly threaten that precious central organ, the body's largest gland that performs an astonishing number of functions that are essential to life.

If you were to take samples of subcutaneous and interior fat tissue, place them in separate laboratory dishes, and drip some stimulating chemicals onto them, the interior fat would respond with six times more harmful secretions, such as inflammatory molecules, than the subcutaneous tissue. So this inner fat is not just dormant flab. It makes bad chemicals in the middle of your body, near your most important organs.

Fat cells also produce two hormones, called *leptin* and *adiponectin*. You may not have heard of them, but they do important things. Leptin secretions increase when you start putting on more fat. The hormone delivers a message to your brain to suppress your appetite and speed up your metabolism so you have less hunger and burn up more calories. However, a rising level of inflammatory chemicals disturbs this internal arrangement and makes your body less able to respond to the leptin message. This creates a situation called leptin resistance. As a result, you eat more and add more weight.

Adiponectin works with insulin to push sugar from the bloodstream into the cells for cellular energy production. For instance, it helps muscles burn fat for energy. The level of this hormone falls as visceral fat increases, a situation that contributes to a failing response of the cells to insulin. This insulin resistance is a prelude to diabetes.

The damaging role of visceral fat continues to emerge as a powerful subplot in the overweight epidemic story. In a 2006 study published in the journal *Obesity*, we, along with researchers from Queen's University in Ontario, Canada, showed for the first time that the presence of excess visceral fat represents a significant and independent predictor of death from all causes—meaning an increased risk for a shortened life.

Here are some other striking findings during the last few years:

- A report in the medical journal *Lancet*, based on data involving 27,000 people from multiple ethnicities in fifty-two countries, concluded that individuals' waist sizes are much more significant indicators of heart attack risk than their BMI numbers.

- A Wake Forest University study of more than two thousand well-functioning older adults, aged 70 to 79, indicated that excess abdominal fat could be a stronger risk factor for heart failure than overall obesity.

- A University of California study among 112 older Latinos concluded that visceral fat may be connected to nerve, blood vessel, or metabolic damage in the brain that underlies cognitive decline and dementia.

- A Japanese study showed that individuals with colorectal cancer had a significantly greater accumulation of visceral fat than people without the disease. Earlier studies during the 1990s showed that visceral adiposity increased the risk for breast cancer. In one 1994 study, breast cancer patients had 45 percent more visceral fat than a group of women without the disease.

Men tend to pack more belly fat than women. It's an issue for them throughout life. Women start to catch up after menopause, when it becomes a common complaint. Compared to premenopausal women, postmenopausal women have about 50 percent more visceral fat. The volume of visceral fat increases with age—for both sexes. We aren't certain why this happens, but we think the reasons likely include a slower metabolism from decreased muscle weight and lean body mass, decreased physical activity, and changes in various hormones that occur with aging.

That's the bad news. Here's the good news: a minimum amount of physical activity, with or without dietary changes or weight loss, goes a long way to neutralize this deep visceral fat, and even shrink it. Imaging studies have confirmed this dramatic reduction. Unlike superficial fat, the interior fat is extremely responsive to physical activity. We don't know why, but it is. You have a lot more of the subcutaneous fat than visceral fat. When you trim body fat in general, you lose a greater percentage of visceral fat. For instance, if you drop 10 percent of your body fat, you may be actually reducing the visceral fat by 30 percent. In any case, as the visceral fat shrinks, your waist circumference shrinks. Your clothes fit better. Usually within weeks you will notice a difference, even with minimal activity. But more importantly, as the inner fat zone shrinks, so does the volume of harmful chemicals it spews out.

And here's the bottom line: You can have all the liposuctions in the world to remove your surface belly fat. It may please your self-image, but it does little for your health. A 2004 article in the *New England Journal of Medicine* concluded that liposuction of surface fat does not affect your cholesterol or blood sugar, demonstrating that this layer of fat is not physiologically important. The answer to visceral fat is not liposuction. It's behavior, and specifically, physical activity.

Your Pants Will Fit Better

Vivian, once a sedentary and slightly overweight secretary, enrolled in our exercise course at the Cooper Aerobics Center. At the end of the six-month program, she reported that she hadn't lost much weight but said, "My pants fit better."

Vivian's response is typical of feedback we hear from many other participants. They start a simple physical activity program and tell us that even within a few weeks their clothes fit better. The explanation is that physical activity trims the visceral fat and adds desirable functional muscle.

In one 2006 experiment, Australian researchers tested the effect of supervised exercise on belly fat, using as subjects healthy but sedentary male and female casino employees. The participants did at least 20 minutes of aerobic activity three days a week and at least 30 minutes of strength training twice a week. The results after six months showed no significant effect on weight, but significant reductions in waist circumference and aerobic fitness.

Do You Have Too Much
Visceral Fat?

It's simple to find out how much visceral fat you are packing. You don't need a doctor to tell you. All you need is a tape measure. The box on the next page provides instructions on how to measure yourself.

Too much visceral fat translates to a 40-inch waist and above for a man, and 35 inches or more for a woman.

In our talks with patients and audiences alike, we try to raise awareness about waist circumference. If it's over the line, you should aim for

HOW TO MEASURE YOUR WAIST CIRCUMFERENCE

1. Use a common cloth tape measure.
2. Take off your shirt. Wrap the tape around your abdomen, just above the level of the hip bone, where the circumference is narrowest as seen from the front.
3. The tape should be snug, but not so tight that it presses into your skin. The loop created by the tape around your middle should be parallel to the floor.
4. Measure your waist circumference while breathing out, with the abdomen relaxed.

a 5 to 10 percent weight loss—with physical activity as a prime tool for achieving it. Even if you are obese, a reduction of that order generates wonderful health benefits.

Interest in visceral fat and waist circumference has started to creep out of the medical establishment and reach the dieting industry. Some weight-loss groups have begun including waist measurement as part of their weekly weigh-in procedure.

3

The Healing Miracle
of Movement

All parts of the body which have a function, if used in moderation
and exercised in labors in which each is accustomed, become
thereby healthy, well-developed and age more slowly, but if
unused and left idle they become liable to disease, defective in
growth, and age quickly.

—Hippocrates, the father of medicine

In 1953 Jeremy Morris, a British health researcher, made the first dramatic scientific breakthrough demonstrating the dangers of sedentary
living. He did so by comparing sitting drivers and active ticket-taking
conductors who operated London's famous double-decker buses. The
conductors climbed around six hundred stairs per working day; the drivers sat for 90 percent of their shift. The ticket-takers, Morris observed,
enjoyed much better health and had half as many heart attacks as their
sitting counterparts. Subsequently, he also made similar observations
among other workers. Postmen who walked or cycled carrying the mail,
for instance, experienced fewer heart attacks than sedentary telephone
operators and clerks.

Morris's observations and other similar follow-up studies fifty years
ago were crude compared to the sophisticated analyses we can do today,
but they planted an idea among researchers that there was something
indeed to this thing called fitness. It would still be years, though, before
enough solid science made the case irrefutable that regular activity helps
you live longer and is, by itself, powerful medicine.

Experts Prove
the Power of Fitness

The center's first landmark study on physical fitness and all types of causes of death from illness was authored by our former research director Steven Blair and published in the *Journal of the American Medical Association* in 1989. It was based on 13,344 patients—10,224 men and 3,120 women—who were followed for an average of eight years. The study showed the connection of health and illness to fitness in very strong terms and in a real scientific way for the first time. The data revealed that individuals in the bottom 20 percent fitness ranking were more than 300 percent more likely to die from heart attacks, stroke, diabetes, and cancer during the follow-up period than the 20 percent in the top fitness category (see the chart below). Fitness was measured by a treadmill performance test.

The powerful results contributed to the American Heart Association's decision to raise physical inactivity from a minor to a major modifiable

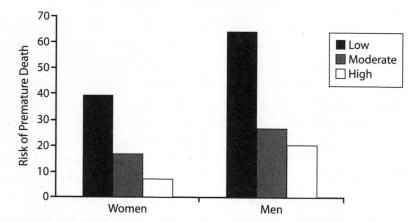

Mortality Rates by Fitness

This graph compresses the findings of our 1989 study into three fitness categories showing the powerful influence of fitness to delay all causes of death. The data reflected more than 110,000 person years of observation (about 8 years per person) following a preventive medical examination, including a fitness test. The highly significant impact of fitness remained intact even after the researchers considered age, smoking habit, cholesterol level, blood pressure, blood glucose level, and parental history of cardiovascular disease. (Source: Blair SN, Kohl HW III, Paffenbarger RS Jr, Cooper RH, et al. *JAMA*, 1989.)

cardiovascular risk factor. Subsequent recommendations from the U.S. surgeon general featured our findings.

In 1995 we took the original findings one step further because some experts had argued that people who are healthy are more likely to exercise than those who are unhealthy. This argument raised a question about cause and effect. A second study examined changes in fitness related to changes in mortality. It involved 9,777 men, all of whom had two medical examinations, including fitness checks, at about a five-year interval. They were then followed for another five years afterward.

The lowest death rate during the follow-up period was among men who were physically fit at both examinations. Unfit individuals who started and sustained a physical activity program between the first and second examinations, and who improved to the "fit" category, had a 44 percent reduced mortality rate compared to those who stayed unfit. These results are illustrated in the graph below.

In 1996 we published another important study looking at inactivity,

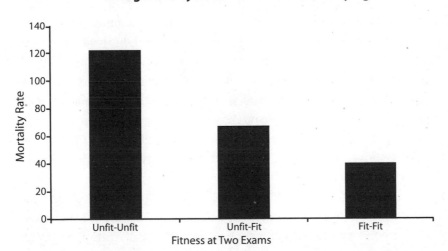

Changes in Physical Fitness and Risk of Dying

This follow-up study, published in 1995, showed that individuals who become physically active and fit significantly lower their risk of premature death. Here, nearly 10,000 men were measured for health and fitness during two medical examinations at five-year intervals, and then followed for another five years. Those who went from unfit to fit between examinations improved their survivability considerably over those who remained unfit. (Source: Blair SN, Kohl HW III, Paffenbarger RS Jr, et al. *JAMA*, 1995.)

smoking, weight, blood pressure, and high cholesterol as predictors of health. The results showed that inactivity was as strong as or stronger than the other risk factors.

The big lesson we have learned from studying data equal to 350,000 patient years at our center is that regular physical activity may be as important as diet and quitting smoking. It will improve quality of life, and quickly, no matter how healthy or unfit you are when you start.

Improve Your Statistical Odds

What do these studies and statistics mean to you?

None of us finishes alive at the end of this adventure called life. The concept of prevention is that you don't eliminate risk altogether—say, of having a heart attack or dying prematurely. Rather, you try to *reduce* the risk. You try to improve your statistical odds, and do the best with the genetic cards you were dealt. People who don't smoke still get cancer, but smokers have a far greater risk. Some people with unhealthy lifestyle habits can live long lives, and some with healthy habits can die young.

Tomorrow is guaranteed to no one. You can follow all the health wisdom in the world and still die young. Doctors can't guarantee patients that lifestyle change will add days, weeks, or months to their lives. But statistically, by following certain behaviors, you increase your longevity. Our research says that however long you have to live, every day of your life will be far better if you are involved in physical activity. Statistically you improve the quantity, and in the process you definitely improve the quality.

Our big database shows what works for large numbers of people, and that boils down to what is most likely to work for each individual patient—and you as well.

Three areas interact with one another in life to influence long-term health: genetics, environment, and behavior. You may be genetically predisposed to a certain illness, such as heart disease. Your genetics may load the gun, but often it is your behavior that pulls the trigger.

Take Claire as an example of how behavior heals in a comprehensive way. She married her college sweetheart, settled down, and started a family. For the next twenty-five years she devoted her time and energy to her children and her husband. In her younger days she had been fit and active, but she failed to take care of herself over the years as she raised her children.

By the time the kids were in high school and college, she found herself chronically drained. She started running out of energy by the afternoon, and by evening all she wanted to do was lie down. Her moods bounced up and down. She was becoming increasingly impatient with both husband and kids, and had developed a disturbed pattern of sleep classically related to stress. She would wake up in the middle of the night and then toss and turn, unable to fall back to sleep again. She was also experiencing stress-related muscle-tension headaches. To make matters worse, she developed abdominal discomfort that was diagnosed as gastritis (inflammation of the lining of the stomach). She began taking medication for her growing assortment of symptoms.

As we monitored Claire and her continuing health problems, we conducted many tests to determine if there were any underlying medical problems that needed attention. We couldn't find any. In time, the likely cause of her problem started to become clear to us: a stressful pace of life and lack of any good cardiovascular conditioning. We felt she needed consistent physical activity and she was getting hardly any. The best prescription we felt we could give her was to counsel her on how to take control of her life once again, and infuse it with the one great healing factor that was missing: physical activity.

Claire followed through. She bought a stationary bike and started pedaling away. She didn't go crazy on it, but she did enough to break a sweat. She called after a couple of weeks and said the few minutes she spent each time on the bicycle felt totally liberating. She was able to reclaim a commitment to herself that had fallen by the wayside while she had focused exclusively on her family. As time passed, she cycled more regularly, and eventually added a bit of light strength training as well. Her program never became excessive. Years later, she's still at it, cycling three times per week along with some light weights, about 45 minutes a session.

The results were remarkable. Her vitality returned and helped her reconnect to her family. She felt better, looked more vibrant, and gradually had fewer and fewer medical complaints. Now she no longer needs medication. On rare occasions, she needs a sleeping pill. Her headaches have lessened significantly, with little need now for painkilling medication. Her gastritis is a thing of the past.

Along with all this, her outlook on life has taken a dramatic upturn. Claire is the perfect example of someone who gradually allowed herself to be pulled away from an active lifestyle, and who, over time, paid the price for it.

In the pages ahead you will see specifically how you can improve your statistical odds against illness and at the same time improve your quality of life—just as Claire did—by working on one simple aspect of behavior: getting physically active. It is not only about the possibility of living longer, but also about living better longer. You'll likely find, as we do with our patients and study participants, that from top to bottom the healing power of movement can be miraculous.

Move to Stop
Metabolic Syndrome

"I feel lousy and that's why I'm here."

The patient sitting on the examination table was a top executive with a major automobile manufacturer. The year was 1995, and the patient was forty-seven at the time.

Dennis's job involved much sitting: at his desk, at meetings, on the plane, and in taxis. Over the years he exercised little and ate too much, mostly on the run. At home, two teenage girls placed great demands on his limited time. For relaxation from the workday stress, he sipped wine, snacked on chips and pretzels, and watched sports on television.

Dennis was too heavy and complained of lagging energy. He had a low level of HDL cholesterol (the beneficial, protective component of cholesterol) along with elevated triglycerides and blood pressure a tad on the high side.

We evaluated Dennis and made recommendations that we felt would alter the teetering course of his health. The most important was for him to engage in some regular physical activity, even if it was just 30 minutes a day of walking.

It was another five years before Dennis returned. He was feeling worse than before. And he looked it, too. He had gotten heavier and sported an expanding belly. He wore size forty-two pants—not a healthy thing for someone under 6 feet tall.

"I tried to do what you told me but something always got in the way," he confessed. "On some occasions I managed to put together a few weeks when I would get out and walk consistently. And I felt better when I did. But something would always come along and derail me. Work, extra travel, family issues. You know how it goes."

For sure, doctors know how it goes. We hear similar excuses all the time.

Dennis's new tests showed that things were clearly worse. He now had evidence of early coronary artery disease. His LDL cholesterol (the "bad" cholesterol that worries most doctors) was not elevated, but his HDL cholesterol was lower than before, and his triglycerides were higher. Moreover, his blood sugar level was considerably higher than it should have been.

At his first checkup, Dennis had had low HDL, elevated triglycerides, and somewhat increased blood pressure. These were the early signs of trouble ahead, and now trouble had indeed arrived. He was developing heart disease and diabetes.

Today, medical science recognizes the particular combination of early signs that Dennis had as a clear warning. They signal the presence of dangerous risk factors with a common cause that most doctors ignore: sedentary living. Simply put, the body doesn't spend enough energy to offset the food calories it consumes. The calories pile up inside. The body becomes heavier and bulges in the middle with unhealthy visceral fat that sends harmful secretions directly into the liver and bloodstream. The fat grows. The muscles shrink and lose their critical ability to burn up calories.

With this metabolic downturn, the body gradually surrenders health and youthfulness, and the ability to withstand stress. The process gets past a certain point, as if passing through a gateway, and then picks up speed in the direction of a killer disease such as heart attack, stroke, diabetes, or cancer.

Whether you pass through this gateway and keep going downhill or wake up at some point and reverse direction requires an individual decision. If we doctors are alert, we can determine a problem in the making, before it develops into outright disease, and give appropriate warnings to patients. And from our standpoint, it is always far easier to prevent the deterioration than to treat the consequences.

Dennis had already passed through the gateway and was developing life-threatening diseases. But he could still keep his situation from going from bad to worse. Pushed by fear, that's exactly what he did. He took responsibility and finally made some overdue changes. In addition to implementing a medical regimen to help control some of his risks, Dennis put himself into a sustained physical activity program and also started to eat better.

The results? His waist shrank by more than 2 inches, his weight dropped by more than 30 pounds, and his fitness level increased from very low to moderate. He felt much better. At his most recent checkup, Dennis's numbers had improved across the board. His lifestyle changes had made a big difference. He was able to make a U-turn and back out of that gateway. Sedentary living had been his ticket in. Physical activity was his ticket out.

You could say that Louise was smarter than Dennis. She stopped right at the gateway and made an instant U-turn.

When we first saw Louise in 2002, she was headed in the same downward direction as Dennis. She was forty-three, was divorced, and had gone through a couple of disappointing relationships. She was depressed and was taking medication. Her blood sugar and triglycerides were up, and she was 20 pounds heavier than when she had started working as a graphic designer fifteen years before.

Louise was very good at what she did. She would spend long hours at a computer doing demanding, eye-straining work, eating fast food at her desk, and returning fatigued to her apartment at mid-evening. With really intense jobs, she might not get home until midnight or beyond. Some days she would sit at her computer for fourteen or more hours.

Louise took our recommendations seriously. She bought herself a step counter and started taking 5-minute breaks throughout her workday. She would walk, first around her office, then up and down the stairs in her building, and even around the block when the weather allowed.

At her next appointment with us in 2003, Louise said she was feeling less depressed and had been able to cut back on her medication. She felt more positive about life and had started to lose a bit of weight.

"I can tell my body shape is changing, because clothes that were too tight a year ago are now loose, particularly around my tummy and tush!" she said.

Tests showed that Louise had indeed made a healthy U-turn. She even talked about taking tennis lessons.

With little fanfare a new health danger has emerged and spread rapidly throughout the U.S. and elsewhere. Dennis and Louise are prime examples. We see a lot of folks like them at our clinic and research facility. They all have a similar set of characteristics. By themselves, these characteristics don't seem so serious. But lumped together, they form a distinct threat. In fact, together they constitute a potentially dangerous condition known as *metabolic syndrome*, which significantly increases your risk of obesity, killer diseases (such as heart disease, diabetes, and

---

WHAT IS METABOLIC SYNDROME?

Your risk for serious illness increases if you have three or more of the five factors below, and probably increases even with only two:

- Your waist circumference is greater than 35 inches for a woman or greater than 40 inches for a man
- Your fasting blood sugar is over 100 mg/dl
- Your triglycerides (blood fats) are over 150 mg/dl
- Your HDL is less than 50 mg/dl for a woman and less than 40 mg/dl for a man
- Your blood pressure is over 130/85 or you need to take a blood pressure medication

Since it was first reported in Italy in the 1960s, this cluster of risk factors has gone by many names, including "the deadly quartet," "syndrome X," "multiple metabolic syndrome," "insulin resistance syndrome," "chronic CV risk factor clustering syndrome," and "Reaven's syndrome" after the Stanford doctor who began reporting regularly about this problem in the late 1980s.

The most accepted and widely used name is *metabolic syndrome*. We believe that this, and all the other names in fact, are misnomers. In our opinion, this cluster of risk factors could very well be called "the physical inactivity syndrome." That's because a sedentary lifestyle contributes directly to each and every element in the cluster.

cancer), physical frailty, and premature death. If you have three or more of the five characteristics described in the box on the next page, you are at very high risk—with quadruple the chance of developing coronary artery disease and triple the chance of developing diabetes.

How widespread is this problem? Fully one out of four adults—and one out of two adults over the age of fifty—develops this set of specific risk factors. By gender, women lead the way, with 55 to 60 percent compared to about 40 percent of men over the age of fifty.

Exceeding the risk threshold puts you into the unenviable company of about 50 million American adults, a number expected to hit 87 million by 2025. Helping to swell the numbers are today's growing population of overweight and out-of-shape kids. One recent survey of two thousand sedentary teens conducted by the Children's Hospital in Boston indicated that nearly a third of them already had metabolic syndrome!

Worldwide, estimates are equally disturbing. The overall prevalence in Canada is estimated at 26 percent, but among Canada's native First Nation peoples, the rate soars to 41.6 percent. In Europe, estimates top 15 percent of the adult population; in Australia, about 16 percent; in the Middle East, 15 to 25 percent.

Metabolic syndrome is clearly an epidemic, and it is recognized as such by medical researchers and public health agencies. But so far it's just a small blip on the public radar screen. Likely you haven't read any headlines about it, seen it featured on television, or heard about it on the radio. And your doctor probably hasn't brought the problem to your attention.

This lack of attention will change soon. Over the last decade and a half, the incidence of metabolic syndrome has skyrocketed. The American Heart Association, the American Diabetes Association, and the National Heart, Lung, and Blood Institute have already issued warnings. The syndrome is a new favorite topic at many major medical conferences. Doctors are starting to get the word.

There are a number of reasons you probably haven't heard about this epidemic:

- Patients typically aren't sick or ailing, even if they have several or more of the risk factors. They don't have hypertension, even if their blood pressure is slightly high. They don't have diabetes, even though their blood sugar is slightly high. And they don't have high cholesterol. Usually they have what we call "watch and wait" values for blood pressure, blood sugar, and cholesterol. They don't know they are already at risk. Right out of the blue they could have a heart attack.

- There is no medication that collectively addresses the cluster of risk factors. Pharmaceutical companies are scrambling to develop such drugs, but have not yet been successful. So none of the big drug makers is beating the drums of public awareness in order to sell a new "breakthrough" drug.

- The public's health attention these days is focused on obesity. Individuals with the risk factor cluster may or may not be excessively overweight. If they are, dieting and losing weight are obviously important for health, but they are only part of the solution.

Prevention and Treatment

Our research clearly indicates that a direct cause of metabolic syndrome in most cases is sedentary living. Our experience also shows that physical activity is one of the keys to prevention and reversal, even for individuals who are overly heavy.

TV WATCHING AND METABOLIC SYNDROME

Do you spend a lot of time watching television or sitting in front of a computer screen? You could be at higher risk for developing metabolic syndrome. That's what two 2005 studies from around the world concluded independently.

In Australia, researchers analyzed the lifestyle habits of 6,241 men and women thirty-five and over and concluded that watching more than fourteen hours a week of TV raised the prevalence of metabolic syndrome, while physical activity lowered the prevalence.

In France, researchers assessed questionnaire responses from 1,900 men and 1,932 women, aged fifty to sixty-nine, about television watching, computer time, and physical activity. Results: most syndrome components increased with sedentary time (TVs and computers) and decreased with higher levels of physical activity. Interestingly, no association was found with time spent reading.

Following is a closer look at the individual risk factors and how physical activity affects them:

Bulging Waistline.   We regard the bulging waistline—packing harmful visceral fat—as the number one risk factor for metabolic syndrome. Research from around the world seems to agree.

If you are sedentary with an excessive waist measurement you can pretty much figure you have metabolic syndrome and are in real danger of developing serious health problems down the road.

Fortunately, visceral fat is extremely sensitive to physical activity. And a little bit of physical activity, we have found, goes a long way in neutralizing and trimming the excess.

People ask us frequently if only fat people, with large waist girths, develop metabolic syndrome. The answer is that many normal-weight people have it as well.

For the most part, people who are fit, even if they are extremely large, don't have an excess waist girth. One of our patients is a former Dallas Cowboys football player who stands 6 feet 8 inches and weighs 280 pounds. He still has a waistline of only 38 inches. This tells us his weight certainly hasn't collected in or around his belly. While most of us don't have builds like professional football players, many of us are built large and muscular, not large and fat. Your waist size can give you a strong hint as to where you stand.

Not everyone who is overweight or even obese has a disease. People may be heavy and healthy. We've said it before and we'll say it again: you can be overweight or even to some degree obese as long as you are physically active. For most people, that's more important than how much you weigh.

Blood Sugar.   In a healthy individual, the body tightly controls the amount of sugar (glucose) in the bloodstream. Sugar is utilized by the cells for energy. When this metabolic arrangement begins to unravel, however, as a result of poor diet and lack of physical activity, trouble is on the way. Doctors consider a slightly elevated blood sugar level—over 100 mg/dl as measured in a blood test—an important indicator of the syndrome and a driving force behind its progression. With a level of 100 to 125 mg/dl you are considered prediabetic. Above 125 indicates actual diabetes, the devastating systemic disease affecting about 15 million Americans.

We regard elevated blood sugar as the other most significant factor in metabolic syndrome. It indicates that your body is not processing blood sugar efficiently, but it is not so bad that you have diabetes. This prediabetic elevation is referred to as *insulin resistance*, a term often used synonymously with *metabolic syndrome*.

When blood sugar goes up, the pancreas responds by producing more insulin, an important hormone that prompts cells to open their outer membranes and allow sugar to enter for energy production. Insulin also stimulates hunger, however, and in excess it contributes to weight gain and extra body fat. The added body fat in turn reduces the sensitivity of the body's tissues to the effects of insulin. As these disturbances gain momentum, the pancreas tries to compensate by releasing still more insulin. Or it may gradually lose its ability to produce sufficient insulin. In any case, glucose (blood sugar) cannot enter the cells. If this scenario goes on for some time, insulin and sugar can rise to toxic levels in the circulation, triggering inflammation, sticky blood, weight gain, and damage to arteries, nervous tissue, and the immune system. These complications are associated with diabetes.

Even a minimum of exercise immediately improves your ability to utilize and normalize blood sugar. A short round of physical activity lowers the blood sugar level for up to forty-eight hours, particularly in individuals with an elevated level. Working muscles generate better blood sugar control, so regular physical activity helps prevent metabolic syndrome from advancing into diabetes.

Cholesterol and Triglycerides.   As determined by a blood test, too little HDL along with an elevated level of triglycerides comprise the third and fourth risk factors. It has been known for a long time that physical activity exerts a beneficial impact on these two indicators of cardiovascular health risk.

HDL protects against the development of heart disease and has been measured and incorporated into routine medical care for years. However, very few medications can increase low HDL, and most have uncomfortable side effects. Fortunately, physical activity does the job effectively.

Triglycerides, which are blood fats used for fuel by the body, appear on routine medical blood tests. Most doctors pay little attention to them unless they rise to extraordinarily high levels, which usually has a genetic basis. Still, even a slightly elevated triglyceride level, a level typically ignored by doctors, indicates that something is amiss metabolically and the body is not functioning optimally. The fats are not being processed, stored, or utilized properly. They build up in the blood, which is not where you want them.

Elevated triglycerides contribute to unhealthy blood vessels and liver dysfunction. We group HDL and triglycerides together because an elevation in the latter causes a decrease in the former. They are intimately linked. Physical activity pushes the HDL concentration up slowly and pushes triglycerides down relatively fast.

Elevated Blood Pressure.   It's well known that physical activity lowers blood pressure in most cases. One session of physical activity has a normalizing effect on blood pressure lasting up to forty-eight hours. Our work at the center shows that physical activity substantially lowers the risk of dying prematurely even for individuals with resistant high blood pressure.

What the Research Tells Us

To be sure, multiple influences—such as genetics, stress, and poor diet—promote metabolic syndrome. But sustained physical activity neutralizes each of the cluster risks and, as a consequence, reduces your chance of later developing a serious disease. With just a little physical activity, your susceptibility decreases, even if the numbers related to particular cluster factors do not improve.

Two studies we did in 2004 make a strong case for our assertion. In one we sampled the medical evaluations of nearly twenty thousand men who had passed through our clinic from 1979 to 1995. They were aged twenty to eighty-three. Of the total, 3,757 already had metabolic syndrome. We had followed up on their individual status until the end of 1996 or until they died. The results indicated that fit men, compared to unfit men, had a substantially lower risk of developing any kind of lethal disease, whether they had metabolic syndrome or not. We also checked to see whether fitness was still a significant protector when body weight was factored in. It was. Fitness status remained protective regardless of weight. The study was published in the *Archives of Internal Medicine*.

The second study, published in the journal *Obesity Research*, set out to determine the presence of metabolic syndrome across different ages and fitness levels in women. About 7,100 women were involved. The results showed a much lower incidence of metabolic syndrome in women with higher levels of fitness throughout all ages. The most striking outcome was the nearly 20 percent incidence of metabolic syndrome among women at the very lowest level of fitness.

In our frequent talks to lay audiences, we warn them about metabolic syndrome. Many of these folks are too heavy and too sedentary, and they know it. Many have tried one diet or another and failed. We consistently get their attention with the fact that this syndrome is really dangerous— something they didn't know about before—and that it threatens their overall health and length of life. Unless they step forward and start moving, we tell them, they are programming themselves for an early death.

> **CLOCK YOUR PROGRESS**
>
> Patients always ask us how fast they can expect to see improvement from a physical activity program. Based on our general observations, you can usually expect the following progress in relation to metabolic syndrome risks:
> - Immediately: blood sugar and blood pressure levels drop toward normal.
> - Within two weeks: triglyceride levels are lower.
> - Within a month: visceral fat shrinks.

What turns them on the most is that they can treat themselves for free with just a little bit of physical activity and sensible changes in eating habits. That's our bait to get them off their rear ends and moving, to get them active on some beneficial level.

Move against Diabetes

Joe, now seventy-one, developed diabetes when he was sixty. He ran a successful business in the steel industry and had always stayed busy, but he was never physically active. He had a family history of diabetes.

Joe had come to our clinic for annual checkups for many years. We followed his health and warned him about his personal risk for diabetes. We saw his blood sugar level creeping up.

Joe was stubborn. He didn't want to exercise or change his diet, and he didn't want to be on medicine.

Every year we would talk to him seriously about diabetes. And every year he would say, "Yeah, I'll do something about it." But he did nothing.

The inevitable occurred. He developed full-blown diabetes with complications typically associated with the later stages of the disease. His coronary arteries began to deteriorate. His immune system weakened. He experienced erectile dysfunction.

In 2005 he was hospitalized with pneumonia. He had an arduous and prolonged recovery. The pneumonia, however, served as a wake-up call. He became scared enough to realize that his behavior was killing him and that he had to make lifestyle changes. He understood he would never enjoy the fruits of his long years of labor unless he did.

For Joe, the struggle continues. While he now keeps his appointments, which in the past he would often postpone, and he's now willing to stay on his medicine, he still hasn't carried out his intention to implement the healthy habits his body so desperately craves. We'll keep working on him. We want him to live to enjoy his grandchildren. Hopefully it won't be too late.

By comparison, consider the example of Ed, a patient of Dr. Janet Tornelli-Mitchell at the center. He was in his sixties, sedentary, overweight, diabetic, hypertensive, with lots of stress from his import business.

Like Joe, whenever Ed came in for a checkup, he said he was trying to eat better, be active, and lose weight, but he just wasn't able to pull it off. It took eight years to get him motivated.

"Listen, this is a game of numbers, like your business," Dr. Tornelli-Mitchell told him after years of hearing the same excuse at his annual examination. "If your business is doing poorly, that means you have to cut your expenses and make more sales. If you are not making money, something is still wrong. It's the same with your weight. You are still eating too many calories and not burning enough. As long as that keeps happening, your problems are going to continue to get worse and I'm going to have to give you more medicine."

The prospect of more medication got Ed to step forward and get off the dime.

"That often motivates people," says Dr. Tornelli-Mitchell. "They are scared of side effects and increased medication. Or when you tell them that they are one step away from becoming diabetic."

Ed started logging his daily diet and physical activity. And every week he reported his progress to a nutritionist at the clinic. Anyone can do the same with a friend or a spouse. Ed's physical activity involved a stationary bike, just a few minutes a day in the beginning. Slowly he graduated to more minutes and eventually he worked with a trainer.

He has lost 30 pounds in two years. His blood sugar, cholesterol, and blood pressure all dropped, allowing his medication to be significantly reduced. Ed feels great and is deservedly proud of himself.

Compare Ed's case with Joe's. Doctors can do just so much, and many patients, like Joe, simply fail to take the responsibility necessary to create and maintain good health. They forget that the healing process begins with their own desires and attitudes.

For us doctors it's always much easier to maintain a patient's health than to restore it after it's lost. When a patient's health deteriorates, maybe we can recoup some of the losses. But not everything is reversible. When you reach rock bottom, which Joe was approaching, you are talking about serious organ damage. Diabetes is a silent killer. It eats away at your body. You don't feel the effects until organs and tissue are destroyed by the toxic effects of high sugar and insulin levels.

The Power of Prevention

Experts think that the massive departure from evolutionary eating and activity habits that we see in today's society underlies the global epidemic of chronic diseases like diabetes. Too much energy-dense food and too little physical activity are taking a big toll.

According to the World Health Organization, 150 million adults have diabetes worldwide, a number expected to double by 2025. In the United States, diabetes affects about 8 percent of the adult population, is the sixth leading cause of death, and is a primary cause of cardiovascular disease, nerve damage, blindness, and premature death. The most common form of diabetes is called type 2, formerly known as adult-onset diabetes, because it customarily affects adults as they get older.

However, the last two decades have witnessed an alarming rise in type 2 diabetes among children. In 2002 the U.S. Centers for Disease Control and Prevention warned that one in three children born in 2000 will become diabetic unless kids start eating less and exercising more. The odds are worse for black and Hispanic children: nearly half are likely to develop the disease.

For each individual the solution is obvious: take action through a healthy diet and regular physical activity before diabetes starts damaging the body. How powerful is this simple prevention recipe? Very powerful, as a group of the country's leading experts concluded in 2002 after a major experiment called the Diabetes Prevention Program. The experiment, conducted at twenty-seven different medical centers, involved 3,234 patients at high risk for diabetes, nearly half of whom were from minority groups at an even higher risk.

The researchers randomly split up the patients, with an average age of fifty-one, into three groups. One group received metformin, a glucose-regulating oral medication for individuals with diabetes. A second group was assigned to at least 150 minutes of moderate-intensity physical activity (walking) per week and a reduced-calorie diet. The third group received written recommendations and annual pep talks on healthy lifestyle, as well as a placebo pill to take twice daily. The latter group served as a comparison for the effectiveness of the other programs.

After nearly three years, the data showed that the second group—following a combined physical activity and restricted-calorie program—had 58 percent less incidence of diabetes than the control group. The results were even more impressive among participants sixty and older, who reduced their risk by 71 percent. What's also striking is that the lifestyle group fell well short of the prescribed walking goal, logging on average only 90 to 120 minutes of walking per week instead of the recommended 150. By comparison, the medication group incidence was 31 percent lower than the controls. The results were similar among men and women, and younger and older individuals.

The aim of this important trial was to see whether either diet with physical activity or the medication could prevent or delay the onset of type 2 diabetes in people already diagnosed as prediabetic. The answer was a resounding yes, particularly for the lifestyle group, and it came so fast that the trial was halted a year early. The results powerfully demonstrated the power of physical activity and diet even among people at high risk for diabetes.

The exciting findings were announced in a 2002 issue of the *New England Journal of Medicine*. The researchers said the trial was strong proof of the ability of lifestyle changes to prevent or delay diabetes in an ethnically and culturally diverse population.

The Muscle-Diabetes Connection

Traditionally diabetes has been regarded as a pancreatic disorder. Research has forced the medical community to broaden that perspective, however, and consider other parts of the body never before thought to be important to diabetes—specifically the muscles.

One could argue that diabetes may be more a disease of the muscles and less a disease of the pancreas.

Muscles are the body's biggest consumers of blood sugar. They gobble it up for fuel like an SUV consumes gas. More important, skeletal muscles store blood sugar. By *skeletal* muscles, we mean the muscles that move your body. The volume of skeletal muscle tissue per body mass is extensive, and thus its storage capacity for blood sugar is quite large.

When you aren't active, your muscles don't use or store glucose in a normal, efficient way. When the muscle cells don't open up for sugar intake, as happens in the prediabetic state of insulin resistance (also known as metabolic syndrome), the sugar builds up in the blood. That's the huge and overlooked connection to diabetes. Unhealthy, inactive muscles can lead to diabetes.

It is not hard to maintain healthy muscles. You don't have to be a bodybuilder. Just by being active and using your muscles, you keep them healthy and efficiently consuming the blood sugar pool. A physically active lifestyle creates better glucose management and a much lower risk of diabetes. You don't get damaging insulin spikes and cellular turnoff to the hormone.

One cardiologist told us recently that she gave step counters to some of her diabetic patients and was dismayed to find out that they were taking on average only one thousand steps a day. That's far too little activity—a formula, in fact, for disaster. We have known for many years that physical activity does wonders for diabetes. Most people with this condition die of cardiovascular disease. But their risk of developing heart disease is directly related to how well they control their blood sugar. Physical activity is the key here. It not only reduces the risk of diabetes, but for anyone with diabetes, it also greatly reduces the risk of complications and prevents premature death.

Rapid Benefits

The impact of physical activity on blood sugar is spectacular. We see changes in days. A person with diabetes who has been sedentary and who implements our minimal physical activity program (Plan A) will

CLOCK YOUR PROGRESS

Based on our general observations with patients, you can usually expect regular physical activity to make the following improvements related to diabetes:

- Within days: blood sugar level decreases.

- Within a month: hemoglobin A1C levels (a measure that doctors use to monitor average blood sugar readings over months) improve.

find blood sugar control changing very quickly. If they aren't alert to this reality, it can be a problem.

We have had diabetic patients come into the wellness program at our center who are taking oral medication and, on occasion, insulin injections. Once they start a physical activity program, many of them need to reduce their medication dosage. Typically, it will soon be too high. If you are a sedentary individual with diabetes and you start a physical activity program, please let your doctor know so your medication can be monitored.

One of our staff workers who joined us in 2004 has diabetes. She hadn't been physically active before, but the work environment motivated her to change. When she went back to see her doctor, after three or four months, he was astounded by the changes he saw and took her off all her medication. She had reversed her condition.

For people with diabetes here's the great news: If you are physically active today, your body will process glucose better the rest of the day, and tomorrow, and even the day after. You get immediate benefit; and if you stay active for the long term, you get long-term benefits. You can practically argue that nothing in the body responds so positively and so quickly to physical activity as blood sugar.

When individuals with diabetes go to their doctor, they typically will get weighed and if overweight, they will more than likely be counseled to lose weight. Studies show that half of them, or perhaps only a quarter, will be counseled on physical activity. This is a gross omission, we believe. The physical activity prescription is sorely underused.

When we speak to medical professionals, particularly to endocrinologists (doctors whose specialty includes the treatment of diabetes), we are constantly surprised by their amazement at how powerful a therapeutic tool physical activity is. They seem to have little knowledge of what a basic physical activity prescription is or what it can do. It appears that they were never trained to have such understanding. That is amazing to us.

Move against Heart Disease

Tedd Mitchell's Story

My family has a troubling history of heart disease. My grand-
father died at fifty-four from a heart attack. My father survived
a heart attack at age fifty-nine in 1987 and then had a coronary
artery bypass, an experience that changed his life.

My father has always been a very busy man. He's an ear
nose and throat doctor. He has always worked hard for long
hours at his hospital and clinic. Until the heart attack, however,
he was never physically active.

After the surgery, he changed. He started eating less. He
bought himself a Schwinn Airdyne stationary bike and began
riding it three times a week at home for about 30 minutes
each session, but never really more because his schedule has
always been jam-packed. He also increased his activity level
by playing golf, something he'd never made time for prior to
his heart trouble. Now he plays golf at least two or three
times a week, getting in a healthy dose of walking with each
round.

Over the course of the next couple of years, he dropped
his weight from 260 to 215, and it has stayed that way ever
since. He lost weight primarily by eating less, and his physical
activity has helped him keep it off.

He is now seventy-nine. We recently did an angiogram to
look at his bypass grafts, and they were all open. He is long
past the time that grafts are expected to stay open like that. He
changed his behavior, and that's what has protected him. Nothing else changed in his life that could account for healthy
grafts after all these years.

As a physician, my father knows good and well the health
reasons for a person to stay active. But if you were to ask him
why he stays active, he will tell you it's because he loves to
play golf.

He had bad bursitis in his hip that bothered him the entire
time I was growing up. His routine sessions on the bike
worked his hip joint without irritating it and strengthened the

surrounding muscles. Over time the bursitis disappeared and hasn't returned. He had cervical disk disease with neck pain. His neck discomfort vanished as well.

The turnaround didn't happen in two weeks. It took a few years. Before his bypass he had accumulated twenty years of muscle and physical deterioration because he was so busy. He couldn't walk a block without some joint discomfort. For years now he has been pulling his own golf cart.

The Power of Prevention

Our research and experience with patients tell us that without a doubt one of the most important things—perhaps *the* most important thing—you can do to prevent a heart attack or stroke is to be physically active. And for patients who already have the disease, it reduces complications. We have seen this great cardiovascular benefit time and time again for both men and women of all ages. Our research has often been quoted by government health agencies as well as the American Heart Association, which in 1992 declared physical inactivity an independent risk factor for cardiovascular disease.

Consider all the traditional risk factors of heart disease: blood pressure, cholesterol, diabetes, smoking, and family history. Depending on which expert you talk to, these factors explain at best 70 percent of cardiovascular disease and at the minimum less than 50 percent. Here's the number one killer disease, and we can't explain a large part of it.

Understanding the role of inflammation in cardiovascular disease has helped fill in some of this knowledge gap. Physiologic and anatomical damage to arteries (called *atherosclerosis*) is now recognized as an inflammatory process. Inflammation of the blood vessels leads to the tissue changes that cause such lethal or disabling cardiovascular events as heart attack, heart failure, and stroke.

Medical science now recognizes a person's level of CRP (short for *C-reactive protein*) as the leading indicator of arterial and systemic inflammation. This substance is abundantly present, and stirring up trouble, wherever inflammatory activity takes place in arterial tissue.

We have found that physically active individuals have a much lower level of CRP than sedentary people do. What's the connection? Physical activity decreases visceral fat, where an array of potent inflammatory compounds is produced, including interleukin-6, which stimulates the liver to make CRP.

In 2002 we checked the CRP level of 722 male patients at our clinic. We found that a clear protective effect resulted from higher levels of fitness. Those who avoided a sedentary, low-fitness status, however, reaped the primary benefit. The same type of protection was seen when we analyzed the data according to weight and waist circumference. Obese and overweight men, even those with waist girth over 40 inches, who were physically active had lower CRP levels than those who were sedentary.

There is also a good deal of data showing that physical activity improves *endothelial* function. The *endothelium* is the vital one-cell-thick inside surface of arteries. This fragile layer produces important chemicals, including nitric oxide that maintains relaxed, dilated, and healthy arteries.

Earlier we discussed how physical activity defuses the components of the metabolic syndrome that add up to increased risk of heart disease and diabetes. Blood pressure, blood sugar, HDL cholesterol, triglycerides, and visceral fat all respond positively.

There are still other ways that physical activity benefits your heart.

It improves blood flow and the inherent health of the blood vessels and the blood itself. If you extract blood from an exerciser and a nonexerciser, the blood from an exerciser flows better through a plastic tube. That's because activity thins the blood. It renders the *viscosity*—that is, the thickness—of the liquid part of the blood more like water than like ketchup. That's how you want it. The better the blood flows, the better it can deliver oxygen and critical nutrients to the cells.

Physical activity also makes red blood cells more flexible. The more flexible they are, the better they flow within the plasma, the fluid part of blood. The tendency for clumping and sluggishness is lessened.

Is physical activity a guarantee that you won't develop cardiovascular disease or suffer a heart attack? Of course not. There are too many factors involved that can trigger disease or even a cardiovascular event like a heart attack, even if you have optimum lifestyle habits.

A stark example of that, even among us big-shot experts, is Steve Blair, our director of research for many years and now a professor of public health at the University of South Carolina. Steve is one of the world's foremost authorities on fitness and health. He has served as senior scientific editor for the Surgeon General's Report on Physical Activity and Health. Steve didn't have a heart attack, but he developed advanced atherosclerosis, and five years ago, at the age of sixty-one, he chose to have bypass surgery. In Steve's own words, "The disease occurred despite my running daily for forty years and being quite fit and eating a healthy diet."

What brought it on despite the fact that research says unequivocally that physical exercise is protective? Steve doesn't know for sure. He thinks it was the stress and sedentary nature of his work.

"For many years I have been working long hours, sitting and doing research and writing at the computer, and I can spend my whole day there, unless I make an effort to exercise," he says. "I also travel constantly, around the world, and frequently don't get adequate sleep. I believe the lifestyle probably caught up with me."

However, Steve is quick to say that he might not be alive if indeed he hadn't made the effort to exercise and follow a good diet.

Move against High Blood Pressure

According to the American Heart Association, high blood pressure killed more than fifty-two thousand Americans in 2003. About 65 million Americans aged twenty and older have high blood pressure—nearly one in three adults. If you have high blood pressure (hypertension), being fit substantially decreases your risk of premature death from cardiovascular disease or other causes. That's the conclusion we made in a 2001 study published in the *American Journal of Cardiology*.

It has been generally accepted that regular exercise helps prevent and reduce high blood pressure. However, the effect of fitness on death rates from cardiovascular disease or other causes among individuals with high blood pressure was not fully understood. That's what we set out to examine in our study.

Using our large database, we calculated and compared death rates for low-, moderate-, and high-fitness categories. We included 15,726 men with normal blood pressure (less than 140/90) and 3,184 men with high blood pressure. They were predominantly non-Hispanic whites and well educated, and had been examined at least once at our clinic before 1993.

The number-crunching produced some persuasive results: higher levels of fitness confer significant protection against death from cardiovascular or other diseases among men with diagnosed high blood pressure.

The details revealed that the death rates among highly and moderately fit men with hypertension were about 50 percent lower than the death rates of low-fitness men with hypertension.

We believe that the results of this study would also apply to women and to other ethnic groups. Indeed, in other reports where we have been able to do parallel analyses for women and men, we find similar associations between fitness and death for both genders.

Physical activity affects high blood pressure in a variety of ways, including lowering stress hormone levels (stress tends to constrict arteries and drive up blood pressure), improving blood fats, improving clotting activity, and preventing insulin resistance.

The primary form of physical activity among the moderately fit group in our study was walking for a total of about 150 minutes a week. Clearly, progressing from low to moderate fitness represents an obtainable goal with some important health benefits for a large segment of the population.

Move against Stroke

In 2002 our researchers teamed up with West Texas A&M University to study physical activity and the risk of death from stroke. We analyzed the medical records of 16,878 men, ages forty to eighty-seven, who had undergone a complete medical evaluation at our clinic, including a treadmill exercise test. When we did the math, the calculations indicated that highly fit men had a 68 percent, and moderately fit men a 63 percent, lower risk of death from stroke when compared to men in the low-fitness category. That's fantastic protection.

Move against Heart Rate Variability

Minuscule beat-to-beat changes in the heart rate are known as *heart rate variability*. They reflect how your body's electrical system responds to the environment. The quicker your system responds, and the more variability between beats, the healthier the system.

Research has shown that individuals with low variability are at higher risk of developing deadly heart rhythms called *ventricular tachycardia* (rapid heartbeat) and *ventricular fibrillation* (disorganized contractions). Both conditions can trigger sudden cardiac death. Patients with these conditions use implantable defibrillators to control such abnormal heart rhythms. People with high variability have a much lower risk.

We recently completed a study with sedentary postmenopausal women showing that only two months of moderate-intensity physical activity can substantially improve the variability of the heartbeat. Thus in just two months you can eliminate a major risk for heart attack in a vulnerable population.

In 2006 Harvard researchers published an analysis of nearly three hundred cases of sudden cardiac death and concluded that regular exercise "may lower the overall long-term risk." That certainly is consistent with our findings. People are better off and safer with consistent exercise than they are with on-and-off activity that strains the body.

Don't Be Fooled by the Stress Test

Starting in the early 1990s, two close friends—one a high school principal, the other a school district superintendent—came through the clinic several times together for checkups. Both in their fifties, they were quite sedentary to start with, had stressful jobs, and ate rather unhealthy diets. Both had developed risks for cardiovascular disease, even though they had passed their EKG treadmill stress test, a basic diagnostic procedure used to determine the presence of coronary heart disease.

We were able to persuade the superintendent to make dietary changes and start a physical activity program, but we never could get the principal to become active, not even minimally, or alter his eating habits.

Several years passed before we saw one of them again at the clinic. It was the superintendent. We asked

CLOCK YOUR PROGRESS

Based on our general observations with patients, you can expect to see the following cardiovascular gains brought about by physical activity:

- Within days: elevated blood sugar level and blood pressure decrease.
- Within two weeks: triglycerides and total cholesterol level drop.
- One to two months: heart rate variability improves.
- Three months to a year: blood becomes thinner.
- Six months to a year: HDL rises.

about his friend and learned that the principal had died of a heart attack a year or so after his last clinic checkup.

The principal never addressed his health issues—his blood pressure, his high cholesterol, his diet, and his activity deficit. And he paid the price. He is a perfect example of someone who develops risks and chooses to ignore them. He also represents a frightening statistic: cardiac arrest is the very first symptom of half the people with heart disease.

You cannot rely on medical checkups or even normal results in tests—all testing has limitations and is not infallible—as a substitute for changing negative lifestyle habits. If you do, you put yourself in great danger.

The principal believed that passing the stress test pretty much meant he was in no danger. The reality is different. A stress test is a wonderful tool for determining serious, obstructive coronary artery disease. It is not so good for finding early disease. You need to have about a 65 percent blockage in your coronary arteries before a treadmill test shows abnormal results. Many heart attacks occur with far less blockage, when arterial plaque ruptures causing an immediate clot. When the clot blocks a narrowed artery, a stroke or heart attack can follow.

We see many patients like the principal who think they are home free because of a good stress test, even if they are sedentary, smoke, and have high blood pressure, a weight problem, and poor blood test results. When you tell them about changing their lifestyles, their eyes glaze over. They're not listening. All they are thinking about is the normal stress test.

Move against Cancer

Chris had it all: a beautiful wife, two children, a house in the best part of town, and a lucrative job in commercial real estate. A former collegiate basketball player, he had been extremely active while young, but by his early thirties his activity had shrunk to an occasional game of pickup ball. By thirty-six he was feeling the effects of ongoing work-related stress and lack of regular activity.

After his checkup at the clinic we had to give Chris some bad news. His evaluation revealed a tumor the size of a golf ball atop one of his kidneys. Fortunately, there was no evidence the cancer had spread.

Chris underwent radical surgery to remove the cancerous kidney and surrounding tissue. Afterward, sitting in his hospital room, Dr. Mitchell had a long heart-to-heart talk with him about the need for some major lifestyle adjustments. Most urgently, Chris needed to defuse the stress in his life and return to some kind of routine of physical activity. The latter would help his health in general as well as reduce the harmful effects of stress.

Chris's brush with death triggered a major shake-up in his life. He left his job and started a smaller, manageable real estate business. The switch gave him more time for both family and physical activities, his two biggest priorities. He now exercises at least five days per week.

It has been ten years since his cancer surgery. There have been no recurrences.

Did the lifestyle changes protect him from recurrence? Perhaps. It doesn't really matter. What does matter is that he has now experienced ten years of quality living that he didn't have prior to his cancer. No one can say that physical activity eliminates cancer, or guarantees you will beat it, but the scientific evidence and individual cases like Chris's sure seem to indicate you reduce your risks.

Move for Prevention

In 1922 two independent studies appeared on cancer death rates among men who worked at different kinds of jobs in Australia, England, and the United States. The researchers reached similar conclusions: rates declined with increasing physical activity demanded by the jobs, and "hard muscular work" apparently promoted cancer prevention. The idea didn't gain traction in the medical community, however, and it dropped from sight for many decades.

In 1989 we published our first major study on physical fitness and all types of causes of death from illness. Based on more than thirteen thousand patients followed for eight years, the report utilized sophisticated scientific methodology for the first time to show a powerful link between all illnesses—including cancer—and a person's fitness level. People at the bottom 20 percent level of fitness were more than 60 percent likely to die not just from heart attacks, strokes, and diabetes, but from cancer as well, compared to people in the top 20 percent.

In 1996 James Kampert, Ph.D., one of our veteran researchers, headed a study on physical activity and cancer mortality alone. The data, based on more than twenty-five thousand men and seven thousand women examined at our center prior to 1989, showed that physically active men had a much lower risk of dying from cancer than nonactive men. The fittest 20 percent of men had a cancer death rate 81 percent less than the least fit 20 percent. Among women, the results suggested a similar, but not significant trend—a weaker finding probably due to a much smaller female sample size. We think that if more women had been included, the results would have mirrored the trend shown by the male sample.

In a later study, our researchers looked specifically at the male database and found that moderate and high levels of fitness were associated with a lower risk of cancer deaths even among smokers.

Following our 1989 study, experts scratched their heads trying to explain the biology of the cancer connection. A search for answers has been going on ever since, and different theories have emerged.

One is that regular physical activity increases the blood flow of natural killer (NK) cells, specific types of white blood cells. Rather than targeting bacteria, viruses, or fungi, they search out cells that look abnormal, such as cancer cells. They search and destroy, and cleanse the body. By increasing the circulation of NK cells, you likely improve your body's detection and destruction of cancer cells.

Another idea involves certain inflammatory molecules produced throughout the body that have the potential to negatively influence the cancer process. Evidence suggests that the more fit you are, the fewer of these molecules you have.

What appears to be at work here is the capacity of the immune system to clean house. Every day we have cells that turn cancerous. The body needs to eliminate them. A sedentary body works sluggishly, including the immune system. That's not a natural state.

We have already discussed the harmful role of excess insulin in metabolic syndrome, diabetes, and heart disease. In cancer, too, we find a connection: too much insulin promotes cancer growth. Physical activity counteracts the excess through the muscle activity that normalizes blood sugar and insulin metabolism. There are clearly some cancers, particularly of the intestinal tract, in which insulin plays a significant negative role.

Another theory is that regular physical exercise helps keeps your body mass down, making if easier to find cancer at an earlier stage.

We have reported also that physical activity reduces the concentration of a harmful substance called *macrophage migration inhibitory factor* (MIF) in obese individuals. At an elevated level, MIF suppresses the gene that suppresses cancer growth.

Some cancers, for instance colon cancer, are more responsive to exercise (see the list below). We believe this benefit is most likely related to lower insulin levels in individuals who are regularly active.

Move against Specific Cancers

I-Min Lee, Sc.D., a member of our Scientific Advisory Board and an assistant professor of medicine at Harvard, is an expert on the role of physical activity in the prevention of cancer. She has analyzed data from studies published in medical journals and found the following evidence of association between physical activity and cancer prevention:

- Active individuals had a 30 to 40 percent reduction in the risk of developing colon cancer compared to inactive people. In general, 30 to 60 minutes of moderate to vigorous activity per day was necessary.

- Physically active women had about a 20 to 30 percent reduced risk of breast cancer. No information exists on the duration of activity needed to produce this effect.

- Those who were physically active had a lower risk of lung cancer.

Lee found no association with rectal cancer, and inconsistent results relating to prostate cancer. Little information exists on the role of physical activity in preventing other cancers, Lee reported; however, a 2005 study of 13,216 women in Denmark found a significant connection between physical activity and lowered risk of ovarian cancer.

Move for Cancer Treatment

There is much evidence that physical activity helps, and helps a lot, as an addition to conventional cancer treatment programs. And interest in it is growing in the medical community.

Here are several conclusions reached by researchers within the last ten years:

- Physical activity may reduce the likelihood of cancer recurrence and enhance survival through its capacity to improve bodily movement, reduce fatigue, and enhance immune function.
- Moderate physical activity reduces relapses and fatigue, and helps patients cope with their illness.
- Physical activity after a breast cancer diagnosis may reduce the risk of death from the disease.

While the benefits of aerobic exercise for breast cancer patients have been fairly well established, University of Minnesota researchers looked into the benefits of weight training and published a positive assessment in 2006. They had hypothesized that increasing physical strength would "reempower" patients psychologically. To test their theory they took a group of eighty-six patients (with an average age of fifty-three) who had been diagnosed with stage 1 or 2 breast cancer. The women were randomly divided, half participating in twice-weekly weight training and the rest serving as a comparison group. After six months, the researchers found that the strength-training group reported significantly higher improvements in their overall quality of life. The improvements were attributed to increased upper-body strength and lean body mass.

Today physical activity is routinely mentioned as a modifiable risk for certain cancers. Those who are physically fit may be less likely to die of cancer or have recurrences. It also appears that physical activity improves a whole spectrum of desirable quality-of-life issues.

Move to Stop Osteoporosis

Jacqueline, one of our patients, is a successful publicist. She's always been very busy in her professional life, but also very sedentary. Her robust health over the years lulled her into believing she didn't need to keep in shape.

As she entered her menopausal years, a series of screenings indicated progressive bone degeneration that ultimately approached the level of *osteoporosis*, a common condition characterized by decreased bone mass and density that causes brittleness and susceptibility to fractures.

"You are not as healthy as you think," we warned her. "You have lost substantial muscle mass because of lack of activity and that is contributing to your bone loss."

Jacqueline had a choice to go on medication to help stem the loss. No way, she said. She had a strong dislike of medical drugs.

The best alternative, we told her, was a physical activity prescription. She had to exercise. And she did. The threat of osteoporosis and medication scared her into forward gear. Jacqueline hired a trainer who tailored a light weight program along with walking on a treadmill for 10 or 15 minutes twice a week. She followed this simple routine, and it wasn't long before she reported that she had lost more than an inch from her waist and dropped a few of her 15 extra pounds. She's content with a low-dose activity program and never became a zealous exerciser; but what is most important, she has stayed with the program. This light activity is basically what she can handle, along with maybe a leisurely walk with her husband on the weekends. Annual screenings have shown that her effort has helped stabilize her bone density and reversed the bone loss process.

Osteoporosis is a multifactorial problem, which includes a genetic component you have no control over. Thyroid and parathyroid diseases can also increase the risk. But there are definitely things you can do to reduce it as well: cut out smoking, avoid excess caffeine, eat a diet with plenty of calcium, get enough vitamin D through sunlight or supplements, and get adequate physical activity.

As in Jacqueline's case, being sedentary is one of the worst things you can do for your bone health. A lack of physical activity reduces bone mineral density and increases your risk of *atraumatic fracture*, a medical term meaning broken bones that are not caused by trauma. People mistakenly think that osteoporosis sufferers take a misstep, fall, and break a hip. However, if your bones are compromised enough, you don't even need to take a misstep. Your hip can break when you are simply standing, and that is what causes your fall. Your risk of fracture from low levels of pressure increases because of osteoporosis. Your mere body weight may be enough to fracture a hip or a vertebra—a reality not widely understood.

The muscle-to-bone connection is also poorly understood. With age we all tend to lose muscle mass, which in turn causes a breakdown of bone tissue. In order to build back bone, you need to build muscle. More muscle stimulates adjacent bone tissue to become bigger and stronger in order to support the additional muscle mass.

A walking program helps to increase your stability and stamina and reduce the risk of falling—extremely important benefits if your bones aren't as solid as they should be. For somebody with poor bone density, a fall is a potentially serious problem.

By itself, however, walking doesn't substantially improve bone mass. You need to engage in some strength training to gain that result, even minimal training, as Jacqueline did. Your best bet for improving bone health with activity comes by directly building up the muscles that support the bone structures.

Sedentary behavior, as we have discussed, often leads to excess visceral fat, and this fat buildup in turn puts your body into a pro-inflammatory state in which the inflammatory chemical interleukin-6 (IL-6) becomes elevated and literally eats away at bones. It poisons bone tissue, specifically the osteoblasts. There are two types of bone cells constantly competing against each other: osteoclasts and osteoblasts. *Osteoclasts* break down old bone tissue, while *osteoblasts* deposit minerals to build new bone. A sedentary lifestyle thus leads to more bone teardown than bone buildup. Over time, the bones become thinner and thinner. Under an electron microscope you can actually see osteoclasts overwhelming the osteoblasts, creating the conditions for osteoporosis.

Most people think of osteoporosis as a woman's disease. Not so. In women, bone density builds up through the thirties, peaks, and then declines. The reversal accelerates during menopause, particularly in the lumbar spine. Afterward, the density still ebbs but at a slower pace. The accelerated drop is due to the hormonal decline of estrogen and progesterone over the span of a decade or so.

Osteoporosis, however, affects men as well. They develop osteoporosis about a decade or so later than women. Bone density declines, sometimes significantly, by the time men reach their sixties. More men, in fact, die of osteoporosis than of prostate cancer.

A few years ago, after acquiring a state-of-the art imaging device (electron beam tomography, or EBT), our clinic started doing routine bone density tests on men over sixty. We were surprised to find how bad the bones looked not just in sedentary patients, but in patients who were aerobically (running or walking) active as well.

Monty, a seventy-year-old attorney, had been a longtime patient of ours, and had always followed an active aerobic program. An EBT scan indicated he had reduced bone density, and follow-up tests confirmed the presence of pronounced osteoporosis. He added a strength-training program to his regimen, and his test results have improved over time. He also takes medication to help the condition.

Through sophisticated scanning we have repeatedly found indications of paper-thin spines and hip bones among many men. We consider ourselves very astute in preventive medicine, but both our clinical and research physicians were surprised by the number of men we otherwise would not have suspected of poor bone density.

These discoveries inspired us to do a study of bone mineral density and fitness, for which there are limited data. In 2004 we reported our findings to the Society for Epidemiologic Research. We took 2,784 healthy, nonsmoking men ages thirty to sixty-nine and measured their fitness via a treadmill test. We then classified them into five levels of fitness according to their age and treadmill capacity. Next we measured their lumbar spine bone density with EBT. In all but the youngest age group (thirty to thirty-nine) we found a strong connection between higher fitness and better bone density. We concluded that increased fitness reduces the odds of developing *osteopenia* (a lower bone mass), which leads to osteoporosis. It is

CLOCK YOUR PROGRESS

Based on our general observations with patients, we see the following bone benefits from physical activity:

• Within weeks: reduced risk of falling because of improved muscle tone and balance.

• Within months: decreased rate of bone mass decline. Increased bone mass requires more intense physical activity and strength training.

important to note that for individuals predisposed to this condition, an activity program must involve not only weight-bearing aerobic activity but strength training as well.

Move to Beat Depression

Mens sana in corpore sano (A sound mind in a sound body).
—Roman satirist Juvenal

Healers throughout the ages have recommended physical activity as a prescription not just for the body but for the brain as well. Only very recently, however, has scientific evidence reached the level where we can confidently say that physical activity indeed protects mental health and should be factored in to treatment plans by doctors.

Marcia first visited our clinic at age forty-eight. She had been through a lot in her life. A car accident at twenty-three had left her with chronic lower back pain, problems with her knees, and cycles of depression and anxiety that sometimes required medication. A demanding job with a real estate company had her constantly on the run and kept her stress level high.

At her initial consultation, we told Marcia about the importance of regular physical activity. She said she understood, but her job always seemed to get in the way. She promised to make a better effort. On a subsequent visit she said she thought her problem was starting some particular program, doing too much and getting overly involved, and then being unable to fit it into her schedule. So she would drop it altogether.

When she was active, however, Marcia noticed the benefits, particularly for her depression. With some guidance from us, she began to incorporate the concept of "less is more." She scaled down the time and intensity commitment to exercise so that it was more practical for her. She found she could stay consistent by walking three days a week and doing some light weight training twice weekly.

The benefits have been both physical and emotional. Her back and joints are far less bothersome with a less intense program, and her anxiety and depression are much more manageable. She rarely needs medication now. Feeling better about herself and life, she was inspired to seek additional fulfillment by involving herself in local charities.

A sedentary lifestyle puts you at higher risk for depression, anxiety, and other mood disorders. Our quality-of-life survey of ten thousand patients shows that clearly: 21 percent of those individuals in the low-fitness category acknowledged having had a significant problem with depression, and another 20 percent had had anxiety. By comparison, there were 24 and 19 percent fewer individuals with those problems respectively among moderately fit patients, and 38 and 33 percent fewer still among the highest-fitness group.

Just exactly how physical activity works to prevent and relieve those mood disorders is a hot field of research. Activity appears to generate a rise and fall in certain mood-governing molecules, promoting countless psychological, neurological, and immune reactions in the body that contribute to both mental elevation and physical well-being.

The most famous of these molecules is the *endorphin*, a morphine-like substance with a painkilling effect produced by the pituitary gland. But endorphins are just part of the reason people feel joy and elation after exercise. Many other biochemical reactions—both short-term and long-term—uplift the brain and mood.

Anxiety and depression have a lot to do with chronic exposure to stress hormones. We doctors like to talk in terms of the fight-or-flight response first described by modern science in the early 1900s. What happens is that the human body produces the same stress hormones in reaction to the chronic pressures and strains of everyday modern life that it did millennia ago when faced with man-eating tigers. These hormones prime you to run or fight. Even though financial worries or a bad relationship with a boss or spouse doesn't require fighting or fleeing (in a physical sense, at least), a constant tide of stress hormones increases your vulnerability to multiple health problems.

Regular physical activity acts as a natural purge for these hormones. Stress-hormone clearance is different in people involved in physical activity than in those who aren't.

After analyzing data from more than thirteen thousand interviews, German researchers in 2004 concluded that physical activity seems to be an antidote for mental distress, depression, and resignation brought on by lost life expectations and major disappointments. An appropriate dosage of activity was a key factor in countering such distress, they added. The researchers found that too little exercise (such as one session a week) has no effect, and "extreme and overly ambitious exercise" may produce an overload of stress chemicals.

Their recommendation: regular aerobic activity, three times a week, to "positively counteract mental distress." The researchers found that life satisfaction reached the highest level for those physically active on a daily basis. Satisfaction with health was also highest among active people of all age groups.

Studies like this provide evidence that as you become physically active, you steer the balance of your nervous system away from the sympathetic side and toward the parasympathetic side. This is an important concept to understand. When you become stressed, the responses in your body become largely regulated by a part of your nervous system called the *autonomic nervous system*, over which you tend to have no direct control. Within this system are two branches: the *sympathetic nervous system*, which primes you to take immediate action, and the *parasympathetic nervous system*, which relaxes and calms you. There are times when obviously you need the former, but you don't want the action juices flowing all the time. Physical activity helps invoke the calming response. It also improves heart rate variability. More variance between beats means the nervous system is reacting more flexibly and efficiently to environmental and mental influences. Depressed individuals have very little variability, an effect frequently observed in patients after heart attacks that can increase the risk of death.

Depression is a terrible, debilitating condition, ranking second behind heart disease for years of life lost due to premature death or disability. It also puts you at a much higher risk of stroke and heart attack. One out of ten Americans will have a depressive episode in their life, and the rate increases among women. Only a small percentage of people with depression—estimated to be as little as 23 percent—seek treatment because of the stigma associated with the condition. And even fewer of them, only 10 percent, receive adequate treatment.

Enter physical activity, shown to be just as effective as medication in alleviating the symptoms of mild to moderate depression. In our big study with sedentary postmenopausal women (discussed in chapter 1), as many as 40 percent of the participants were taking antidepressants when they started. Many told us they had heard that exercise could make them feel better, but they expected us to tell them they had to start

CLOCK YOUR PROGRESS

Based on our general observations with patients, you can
usually expect regular physical activity to make the following mood improvements:

• Immediately: mood
  elevation and a calming
  influence.

• Three months to a year:
  mood stabilization.

jogging five or six days a week at a pretty intense pace. That's not what they heard from us. You can't tell that to a depressed person. We told them that anything they do is better than nothing. You can start with 5 minutes of walking. Two weeks down the road you can increase the time by a few minutes. Four weeks later add more minutes. Pretty soon you're up to 15 or 20 minutes and then a half-hour, and along the way you are getting some physical benefits. You just ease into it.

Treating depression with medication, while necessary in many cases, is also a double-edged sword. You alleviate the symptom temporarily, but side effects can be substantial and the pills are expensive. People tend to not stay on the program and to stop taking medication within six months. Physical activity, on the other hand, makes you feel better, healthier, and happier.

To be sure, depression is complicated and we would be amiss in saying blithely that physical activity represents a simple solution. It works well in many cases, but in others, as we will describe in a moment, the physical and mental drain of depression produces paralyzing negativity and apathy.

We have learned from patients that physical activity quickly reduces anxiety. We haven't done formal controlled studies to confirm this claim, but our impression is that it acts short-term as effectively—and much more safely—as a tranquilizer.

According to Michael Landers, an expert at Arizona State University on the subject of exercise and mental health, the impact on anxiety reduction is as follows:

• Best results are with aerobic exercise.

• Results are best after weeks of regular exercise.

• Best benefits go to those of low fitness to begin with.

• Best benefits go to those high in anxiety to begin with.

Lifting a patient out of depression with a simple prescription of physi-

cal activity is tremendously gratifying for our doctors at the Cooper
Aerobics Center. It's not always so
easy to pull off, though, especially
in cases of serious depression. Janet
Tornelli-Mitchell is one of our staff
doctors, and two-thirds of her
patients are women. She frequently
encounters patients with significant
depression. She explains:

"These are women who tend not
to be the healthiest or who don't
take good care of themselves. They
may have low self-esteem, perhaps
were abused at one time or another
in their lives. Sometimes they have
marital difficulties or a husband
running around. They are stressed,
irritable, and anxious. They sleep
poorly and lack energy. They are
caught in a vicious negative cycle,
and overeat from stress. They get
heavier and heavier.

"Their emotional burden drains
so much of their energy and time.
With this state of mind it is practically impossible for them to
become physically active, follow a
dietary plan, or achieve a goal of
better health. Trying to do so usually ends in failure. The effort simply stresses them out even more.

DOCTORS JANET AND TEDD MITCHELL: PARENTS AS MOOD MODELS

"Our kids are teenagers and have grown up in a house where both parents talk enthusiastically about health and fitness. Kids are kids, of course, and they are going to roll up their eyes when parents go on about something like healthy lifestyle. So we try not to nag them about exercising. They do see us, however, practicing what we preach.

"Recently, our fifteen-year-old daughter became upset because of a row with a friend. She told us what had happened and announced that she was going for a jog. She came back and was a different person.

"For sure, it's not a foolproof strategy, but we believe in trying to be models for our kids and leading by example. If you see your child down and depressed and worried, how do you reach out? If you yourself are into a physical-activity routine, you know that physical activity can help, so you may be able to inspire your child to get up and take a walk with you. It's a good way to help a loved one and yourself at the same time."

They might put on a step counter, but not give a hoot whether or not they can reach their goal, and likely not have the energy for it.

"Patients like this are difficult to treat. How do you help them break the vicious cycle and make positive lifestyle changes? The answer is that you often can't do it without first getting to the root of the depression with a combination of skilled therapy and medication. These are times when we have to put on hold the good lifestyle prescriptions for physical activity and diet.

"You have to first overcome the emotional barrier even to get them into a minimal program. That's my experience with hundreds of women like this. A minimum program can certainly help the mood. The hard thing is getting someone with a serious depression disorder to do it. It is much easier if the depression is mild or moderate, and then the physical activity indeed has a good effect."

Move to Overcome PMS

Many studies show that premenstrual symptoms (PMS), including depression, irritability, and mood swings, can be improved by physical activity.

Again, Dr. Janet Tornelli-Mitchell's feedback from her experience with patients provides helpful perspective: "My female patients who go from a sedentary lifestyle to even a low level of physical activity tell me consistently that their PMS improves.

"Take Sandy, twenty-five, recently out of college, on her own, and trying to find a job in New York. She always experienced some crankiness before her period but her move to the big city stressed her out in a big way. Initially, her PMS was worse. In New York, however, she did a lot of walking. Much more than she had done in Dallas, her home town, where she drove a car to get around. It wasn't long before she noticed that she wasn't as moody and emotional before her period despite the fact that she was still under a lot of stress.

"Alice, a patient in her forties, had a similar experience after being transferred by her company from Austin to Paris. Paris is a great walking city and Alice walked a good deal, including to and from work, much more than she ever had before. Over months, her clothes got looser and she started to lose weight. At first she wondered if something was physically wrong with her. But soon she realized that she was feeling better, had more energy, and was less moody around the time of her period. Her walking activity was creating a higher state of well-being. She didn't eat as much as before and wasn't as hungry. Alice was in

Paris for three years, and then was transferred back to Austin, where she resumed her previous sedentary living. She drove back and forth to work, rediscovered Oreos, started to overeat again, and her physical status regressed. Happily, she realized what was happening, launched into a physical activity program, and reversed the process."

Move for a Better Memory

At our clinic we monitor patients over the course of many years. An observation we've made is that those who remain active physically do better mentally. One of our patients, a gentleman in his eighties, finds time to walk every single day. He heads a jewelry company and is in full charge of day-to-day operations. We see no decline in his function.

The aging process tends to slow mental function a bit, but seniors we see who are fit appear to experience less decline than their unfit counterparts.

Research confirms our observations. In 2003, for instance, doctors at the University of Washington recruited 154 Alzheimer's patients to see if physical activity could make a difference in their lives. These were all patients receiving standard medical care at home. Half the patients were randomly chosen to do at least 60 minutes of physical activity a week—a minimum by any standard. But just this bare minimum resulted in greater physical functioning and less depression within three months.

After two years, the researchers found that the physically active group continued to have many improvements compared to the nonactive group, which continued to deteriorate. Moreover, there was less institutionalization due to behavioral disturbances among the active group.

In another study, these same doctors found that regular physical activity three times a week or more—compared to fewer than three times a week—significantly reduced the incidence of dementia and Alzheimer's among a population of 1,740 individuals over the age of sixty-five. The subjects were monitored for about six years. The researchers concluded that regular physical activity produces a "delay in onset" of age-related cognitive disorders, "further supporting its value for elderly persons."

Two large studies in 2004 showed very clearly how good an effect physical activity has on mental function over long periods of time. In the first, Harvard researchers analyzed questionnaire and telephone interview responses from sixteen thousand women over a nearly twenty-year time span. They found a 20 percent lower risk of mental impairment among women who reported the most physical activity, including walking, compared to those who reported the least amount. The most active individuals scored much higher on tests measuring learning, memory, and attention. The women were in their late fifties and early sixties when the study began, and in their seventies and early eighties when the final comparisons were made. "Being active does protect your brain," said Jennifer Weuve, the lead researcher.

The other impressive 2004 study, involving more than two thousand men (ages seventy-one to ninety-three), took place in Honolulu. The researchers compared minimum walkers (less than a quarter-mile a day) to maximum walkers (more than two miles). Over a nine-year period, the former group turned out to be about twice as likely to develop dementia, including Alzheimer's, than the longer walkers.

Studies of mice also support the idea that physical activity can help a person's mental function as he or she gets older. A 2005 study in the *Journal of Neuroscience* reported that regular physical activity stimulated the production of neurons in the memory sector of the brains of older mice—the equivalent of about seventy in human age. After just one month of exercise on a running wheel, they were able to learn new tasks better than sedentary mice. Previous research had shown the same result in younger mice.

"I would absolutely recommend people exercise for the mental benefits—especially the elderly," Henriette Van Praag, a staff scientist at the Salk Institute for Biological Studies in La Jolla, California, where the mouse studies were conducted, told the *Los Angeles Times*. "People don't care about whether they're a size four or a size six as they get older. But they do care where their car keys are and whether they'll have the ability to play their card games and enjoy life."

In the study, Van Praag explained, "the sedentary mice barely learned the task at all. The aged runners were almost as good, if not better, than the young sedentary mice. It was almost a reversal of mental decline."

While it was not a human study, the revelation that new neurons can be formed later in life—a process called *neurogenesis*—is a major and exciting finding. Scientists previously had believed that we lose nerve cells, and don't gain more, as we age.

We know that physical activity helps mental performance in a number of ways. It increases oxygen flow to the brain, which may contribute to new blood vessels that in turn contribute to the growth of new cells. It stimulates growth factors, including one called *brain-derived neurotrophic factor*, important for the survival of new nerve cells. Finally, it boosts *neurotransmitters*, brain chemicals such as dopamine and serotonin, that are involved in cognition.

Our simple advice is that, along with physical activity, do something that actively engages the memory. Instead of just watching TV, read a book. Do crossword puzzles. Neurologists also recommend that you try to learn new physical tasks such as brushing your teeth with your left hand if you are right-handed. Brain scans show that doing things that our bodies are not used to doing physically stimulates high brain function.

Move for More Energy

Grandma Estelle always takes her extended family on annual vacations. One year she took them to Hawaii, but instead of having a good time, she became depressed. She had become increasingly aware that a chronic lack of energy prevented her from participating in the fun things that other family members did, such as taking hikes, bike rides, and long walks on the beach. She was too far out of shape. A little effort would exhaust her. Although she was on vacation with loved ones, she found herself alone much of the time, watching TV just as she did at home.

After a lecture from us during a medical checkup, she decided to do something about it. Back home, she launched into a simple program of physical activity every day, beginning by just walking around her house. She gave up a bit of TV every day and instead started using her house as a playground. It was enough to raise her in a very short time out of her sedentary rut and into better physical shape.

The next vacation was much different. She was out there, maybe not leading the pack or going the whole distance, but happily participating and able to generate enough energy to have some active fun. Just by putting a little movement in her life, she was able to grab a whole lot more of life.

Henry started coming through the clinic for medical checkups about fifteen years ago. He's a retail executive who over the years has worked hard, poured his energy into his work, and then come home to watch a lot of TV. He never exercised. He was way out of shape. He was typically sedentary.

We could never get him to change his ways despite constant nagging. But his youngest daughter provided the spark—indirectly. When she got to high school, she decided to try out for the drill team. However, she previously had been very sedentary, as a lot of kids are, and had put on considerable weight. She failed to make the team.

Henry decided to help his daughter make a successful try the next time by developing a physical activity program for her and participating in it himself to encourage her.

Henry's daughter never did make the drill team. But by getting involved, Henry accomplished a breakthrough for himself. He got off the couch and onto the sidewalk. He started walking in his neighborhood about five or six times a week and now feels energized in a way he hasn't felt for years. His previously worrisome medical test scores also show the influence of sustained physical activity. A father's concern for his daughter's well-being became a blessing for his own health.

The quality-of-life survey we did for this book, analyzing the responses of ten thousand patients to specific questions, shows pretty clearly that physical activity is a great energy booster. Among low-fitness patients, 26 percent said they had had a significant problem with unexplained fatigue. Among moderate-fitness patients, only 16 percent had had a problem. In the highly fit category, only 11 percent of patients had ever been troubled by fatigue.

Sedentary living robs you of energy. Physical activity brings it back and reduces fatigue. It's as simple as that. On the surface you might think it would work the opposite, that activity would make you more tired. If you think that way, you are buying into a persistent myth. As we have seen, physical activity makes all the body's systems operate better, from top to bottom. As a by-product, your body generates more energy.

We find that sedentary patients who come through our clinic have learned to live with lower and lower levels of energy. For them fatigue has become habitual. And one by one, the little things and tasks in life that they did before have disappeared. It's always interesting to us as doctors that they rarely see themselves as being fatigued. They have become so accustomed to it. They often attribute it to the attrition of life. To us it's more of a loss of life that is so preventable. Our bodies are made to be used. If we don't use it, we lose it.

CLOCK YOUR PROGRESS

Based on our observations with patients, within days you can usually expect a stepped-up physical activity program to start generating more energy and improved capacity to carry out everyday functions.

From the time we hit our thirties, we go physically downhill unless we stay physically active. Patients frequently tell us that the same things they did when they were thirty are now much harder to do at forty. They need to expend more energy. They'll say, "Well, heck, I'm forty." Or, "Heck, I'm fifty, and this is the way I should feel. I work long hours and I can't expect to do now what I did at twenty-five."

What always surprises them—and gratifies us as physicians—is that when they start getting consistently active, the energy returns and their everyday life starts perking up. They start regaining the strength and energy to do things they did before.

Beyond the common type of fatigue that many sedentary people experience is a persistent and profound condition often accompanied by sore throat, muscle and joint pain, headache, and impaired concentration and memory. We called this *chronic fatigue syndrome*. People in this situation have a reduced level of physical activity, resulting in cardiovascular and muscular deconditioning, which compound their symptoms.

Researchers at the Royal Liverpool University Hospital in England recently demonstrated that an exercise program, added to standard treatment, improved physical functioning, sleep, disability, and mood among these patients. The exercise was tailored to each patient's functional abilities. The gains were substantial compared to other patients who received only the standard care. Nearly 150 patients were involved in the yearlong study.

The researchers noted that before the start of the study, only 15 percent of the patients believed that their illness was related to physical deconditioning. At the conclusion, 82 percent realized by their own personal improvement that there was a connection.

Move for Better Sleep

"I don't sleep well at night, doctor. Can you give me a pill?"

Doctors hear this request repeatedly, and often will write out a prescription for a grateful, sleep-deprived patient. Taking a pill may be a simple remedy for many; however, there is a price to pay. These best-selling drugs produce mental impairment, daytime sleepiness, increased falls and fractures, and depressed mood. With them, you may be in bed and asleep for eight or nine hours, but you are not getting a night of restorative sleep.

There are many reasons people can't fall asleep. One usually overlooked reason is lack of physical activity. If you are sedentary by day, that often translates to disruptive sleeping patterns at night. You sleep lighter and don't spend as much time in the restorative stages as normal.

Keep in mind that nature is based on cycles of rest and activity. If you don't get enough of one, the other is affected. Without enough activity, you have more difficulty initiating and maintaining sleep. Physical activity quickly improves both, and recognition of that has made it a primary remedy at sleep clinics.

Anxiety and depression are two major causes of poor sleeping patterns, and physical activity helps defuse both.

In our quality-of-life survey at the Cooper Aerobics Center, we found that 29 percent of sedentary patients had a history of insomnia. Among individuals at the moderate fitness level, the incidence was 25 percent. For highly fit patients, the incidence was 22 percent.

Sedentary patients often complain of insomnia. Among them are quite a few intense type A people, individuals who are very busy but not physically active. They will rationalize their insomnia away, saying, "I don't get a lot of sleep and I don't seem to need it. It's not a problem."

A typical conversation in the clinic will go like this:

"How many hours do you get?"

"Maybe five or so. And it's about all I need."

"How do you feel during the day?"

"Well, I'm not as energetic as I used to be, but I'm okay."

They don't appreciate how good they can feel until they start a physical activity program and soon experience a higher level of energy and better sleep. They often share their amazement at the difference.

Ken, a former government official and now a busy attorney, was a typical type A patient. He always needed sleeping pills. But after having cardiac bypass surgery years ago, he turned his life around. Among other things, he got physically active. As a result, his sleep pattern improved. He travels constantly on behalf of his law firm; nevertheless, he sleeps better, without the need of sleeping pills, and feels more energized.

The benefits didn't stop there. His allergies improved—a huge problem for him before—as a result of his immune system operating at a higher level. Previously he had been on gastrointestinal (GI) medications, and had had surgery for a bleeding ulcer in the early 1980s. His GI tract now works better as well, without any medication.

For activity, Ken favors the treadmill. On nearly a daily basis, he climbs on his treadmill at home, switches on the television, and zones out from the cares of the day.

Sleeping well has a great deal to do with energy. Instead of waking up with the battery 75 percent or less charged, you wake up fully charged. Patients often tell us that their quality of sleep improves with physical activity. They fall asleep faster and experience more restful and restorative sleep.

In our quality-of-life survey, we also asked patients whether they ever had had a significant problem with snoring. Fully one-half of the patients in the sedentary, low-fitness category answered yes. Compare that to moderately fit individuals with 35 percent, and the highly fit group with 22 percent answering yes.

Jim is a good example of how physical activity can often remedy a disturbing snoring problem. Although happily married, he and his wife, Virginia, slept in different rooms. She couldn't stand his loud, relentless snoring—an affliction shared by perhaps 30 percent of men and 19 percent of women in this country.

Jim, a successful lawyer, came to see us at the insistence of Virginia. He was forty-seven and felt basically healthy for his age, but he had become totally sedentary and was about twenty pounds overweight.

CLOCK YOUR PROGRESS

Here's how quickly physical activity will help your quality of sleep.

- Within days: better, restful sleep.
- Three months to a year: reduced snoring and need to awaken at night to urinate.

During his initial evaluation we discovered evidence of coronary artery disease. He had, in fact, the coronary artery system we would expect to see in a man twenty years older.

We discussed the implication of his cardiovascular situation and proposed a remedial plan. Jim immediately committed himself to make some necessary lifestyle changes.

Within a year he returned to the clinic for another evaluation. He was a changed man. He had implemented a consistent program of physical activity, going from initially walking to light jogging several times a week for 40 minutes at a time.

Steadily his fitness level increased and the extra pounds melted away. The activity program, along with medication, helped improve his cardiovascular picture significantly. As for the snoring, the decibel level went way down, and Jim and Virginia were able to share the same bed again.

Though physical activity can help you sleep better, it is important to fit it into your schedule properly. Here are two important no-no's we share with patients regarding their exercise schedule:

1. Don't cut into your sleep to get up earlier to exercise. Adjust the rest of your day to fit the activity in. People who have disruptive sleep patterns, from either not enough sleep or not the right kind of sleep, tend to produce less leptin, a hormone responsible for appetite suppression. Lower leptin could result in staying hungrier during the day and gaining weight as a result. Sleep deprivation may thus contribute to overeating, particularly sweets and carbohydrates. Ask any doctor. We all vividly remember the sleep-deprived days of internship and residency and all the doughnuts, pizzas, and sodas we filled ourselves up with.

2. Don't exercise before bedtime. Evening exercisers have more trouble falling asleep. You put your body into a physiologically excited state that makes it harder to settle down.

Move for Better Sex

Marv is a very successful fifty-six-year-old who climbed high on the corporate ladder at a large company. He is well educated, with an advanced degree in engineering. You would think that a smart man like

Marv would understand the importance of regular physical activity. But not so.

Marv charged into the corporate life right out of graduate school, determined to make his mark. Three decades later he realized that his "nose to the grindstone" mentality hadn't been so hot for the rest of his body. He was totally sedentary, weighed more than 300 pounds, and felt lousy.

At the time of his first evaluation in 2001, we were concerned about worrisome risk factors such as high cholesterol and high blood pressure. Marv understood the importance of controlling his health risks, but he was most anxious about the downturn in his love life. He had become impotent, and this was the major reason he came to us for help.

Marv listened to our recommendations and left determined to change his life. He now applied to his lifestyle the same determination that had brought him success in his career. He immediately started a walking program. He reported a couple of months later that he was feeling not only more energetic, but happier and more affectionate, which was all translating to an improved sex life.

Marv did well for several years. But about four years later he was sucked back into long hours at work and found no time for physical activity. His fitness declined, and with it his erectile function.

Marv returned to the clinic, reassessed himself, and left with renewed determination not to lapse into inactivity. When we heard from him last, he was regaining his stamina once again.

Marv's individual experience is indicative of our general observations with patients. In our quality-of-life survey, we asked male patients if they had ever had a significant problem with impotence. Keep in mind, these are patients of all ages. About 10 percent of the low-fitness group answered yes. Slightly more than 7 percent of moderately fit individuals answered yes. Among individuals in the high-fitness category, 4.6 percent said yes.

We also asked both male and female patients about decreased sex drive. For the low-fitness category, 30 percent said they had had a significant problem. Among the moderately fit, the percentage was 22. In the high-fitness group, the lower incidence was under 20 percent.

Finally, we asked patients if they ever had had significant sexual problems. The question was deliberately vague because people define sexual problems very differently. A problem for one man or woman may not be an issue for another. We posed the question so that the patient could answer according to his or her idea of what's problematic. The results: low-fitness category, 11 percent said yes; moderate-fitness, 7.4 percent said yes; and high-fitness, 5 percent said yes.

From our observations, a sedentary lifestyle diminishes sexuality and the function of your sexual organs. Physical activity helps maintain or restore your sex life. There are several parts to the equation here: human relations, sex drive, and sexual function. All are independent factors.

Physical activity doesn't really contribute to the human relations part, except if you like to participate in group recreational activities where you might meet someone of interest. Studies do show, however, that people who have finished working out appear to be more receptive to the idea of participating in sex. It's an immediate thing. And physically active people also tend to feel better about themselves. The better self-image, too, connects with a greater likelihood to pursue an active sex life.

Physical activity for sure helps support the body's internal machinery involved with sex drive and function. Sex drive depends on hormones. The sex drive hormone in both men and women is testosterone. One ingredient needed to increase testosterone circulation is physical activity.

Moreover, physical activity raises blood flow. Our sexual organs—both male and female—are blood-flow dependent. If you don't get adequate blood to your private parts, they don't function as well as they should. The male connection with blood flow is better known, and receives more attention because of the erectile dysfunction problem. But it is every bit as important for women, where good blood flow is critical for clitoral function and hormonal secretions. Without good blood flow, a woman will tend to have vaginal dryness and painful intercourse.

Anatomically, physically active individuals tend to have more flexibility of the pelvic muscles and less complicating conditions that impair the sexual act, such as lower back pain and hip disorders. The sex act involves physical labor. If you are so deconditioned that you can't do the work, having desire and a sex drive may not do you any good. If you are a sedentary male, Viagra may not rescue you. Viagra will take care of the erection, but not the peripherals. Moreover, if you are way out of shape, strenuous sex could put you at cardiovascular risk. In other words, it could be the last thing you do.

One of the more interesting recent studies done on the connection between physical fitness and sexuality was conducted by Stanford University aging expert Walter M. Bortz II. Bortz set out to identify behaviors that might improve sexuality among people fifty years and older. He sent a questionnaire to the membership of the Fifty-Plus Fitness Association, a group of about two thousand individuals nationwide who share a common interest in the health effects of a physically active lifestyle for older people. Members range in age from fifty to ninety-four years (average age: sixty-two). Their most popular activity pursuits are walking, cycling, and jogging.

> **CLOCK YOUR PROGRESS**
>
> Here's how quickly physical activity can help your sex life:
> - Within days to weeks: sex drive increases.
> - Six months or more: improved circulation improves sexual organ function.

Bortz asked about their frequency of episodes of intimacy per week. That included intercourse, kissing, hugging, and massage.

The results indicated that higher levels of fitness promote sexual intimacy. Among women, one or more episodes of intimacy per week were reported by 30 percent, 38 percent, and 66 percent for the least, middle, and most-fit groups, respectively. Among men, the numbers were 46 percent, 60 percent, and 63 percent.

The membership of this association boasts a considerably lower incidence of early death compared to inactive groups. Bortz suggests that increased sexuality may be part of the life-span equation, and he encouraged doctors to ask about sexuality when taking medical histories of older people. A program of physical activity may be a "valuable prescription," he concluded. "Physical fitness and high levels of sexual activity are mutually supportive elements of successful aging."

Move for Better Digestion and Elimination

A sedentary lifestyle fouls up your digestive and elimination machinery, leading to increased reflux, indigestion, heartburn, constipation, bloating, gas, and abdominal pain. Although we don't clearly know the precise mechanisms involved, we do know that physical activity protects and improves intestinal operations from top to bottom. Here are a few reasons why:

- Decreased transit time. From the beginning of the GI tract in your stomach to the very end of your colon, physical activity speeds things along. You want food to be processed efficiently and the waste products to move quickly through the system. If wastes move slowly, they start dehydrating and compacting, making them harder to eliminate. You don't want those toxic residues loitering in your body. The less exposure you have to them, the less your risk of colon cancer is. Research has clearly shown that physical activity reduces the risk of colon and pancreatic cancer.

- Improved overall circulation, including circulation to the intestinal tract. This benefit reduces or reverses a disorder of the blood vessels that feed the gut called *intestinal angina*. The symptom is cramping pain after eating, a result of feeble blood supply to the intestines. Not enough nutrients and oxygen are being supplied to the intestines to enable the tract to do its job of food breakdown and absorption. This condition is the intestinal version of cardiovascular angina, where not enough blood supply reaches the heart muscle.

- Improved nerve supply. The intestinal tract contains a great deal of nerve tissue to generate the physical action (motility) and the countless biochemical reactions involved in food processing.

- Improved immune function. The digestive tract is home to about 70 percent of your body's immune system activities. A healthy intestinal tract helps to protect you from infections and disease.

Move against Heartburn

In our quality-of-life survey, 51 percent of low-fitness patients said they have had a significant problem with frequent heartburn. Of the folks we categorized as moderately fit, 22 percent had a problem. In the high-fitness group, only 12 percent answered yes. That means 67 percent fewer people in the moderately and highly fit group suffer from heartburn, compared to individuals in the low-fitness group.

There are medical subtleties between reflux, acid indigestion, and heartburn, but patients understand—and experience—these problems simply as heartburn. As you can see from our survey, a substantial number of sedentary patients complain of heartburn. They have generally spoken to their family doctor about it, and when they see us, they are taking Nexium or some other antacid pill. It works fine for them, and they usually have no need to see a specialist.

What they don't know, and what we tell them, is that if they get physically active, their gastric emptying time improves. The stomach does its job better and faster and pushes the food down into the intestinal tract. Excess acid doesn't sit around in the belly longer than it needs to. Physical activity streamlines the operation by enhancing gastric emptying. As you lose the mass of the food quicker due to more efficient processing, you have less food bulk mired in your middle. Otherwise, when you lie down with all that weight in the middle, there's more pressure on the gut, forcing the acid upward into the esophagus. The equation is quite simple: less central bulk = less pressure = less heartburn.

Over the years we have found that many patients start putting on extra weight as they get increasingly inactive. They didn't have heartburn before. Now they have it, along with the 5 or 10 pounds of visceral fat filling their midsection.

The pill a doctor gives you to relieve the acid production doesn't get to the root of the problem. Before you try a pill, try physical activity. Get your weight down by 5 or 10 pounds. It turns out that both physical activity and weight are independently predictive of heartburn. Fitness helps the problem regardless of weight, and weight loss helps regardless of fitness.

You're not doomed to live with heartburn. It doesn't come with age. But it often comes with fat. So we try to get people active, and often they don't need the medication as a result. We hear it over and over again from patients who have gotten active. They tell us they don't remember the last time they had to take Tums or Nexium.

Move to Beat Constipation

Have you ever had a significant problem with chronic constipation? That was one of the questions we asked the ten thousand patients in our quality-of-life survey. We were surprised by the results. There was hardly a difference among the different categories of patient fitness. For the low-fitness group, 7.2 percent answered yes. Moderately fit, 7.6 percent. Highly fit, 7.2 percent.

Constipation turned out to be the single negative exception in our analysis of the impact of physical activity on quality of life. We had expected to see a powerful association, but were surprised, first of all, by the relatively small percentage of people complaining about constipation. Although sedentary patients, in particular, frequently tell us in reply to a direct question that they do not have daily or regular bowel movements, the issue of irregularity for many people apparently doesn't equate to a constipation problem worth noting in the questionnaire. For them irregularity is a normal thing.

From our years of clinical experience and patient feedback, we find that regular physical activity clearly makes you regular. Physical activity stimulates the activity of the intestines, the motility of food and subsequently of wastes. Physicians are well aware that constipation often accompanies prolonged bed rest and immobility. When ambulatory hospitalized patients can't poop, doctors tell them to start walking the halls.

The connection between sedentary lifestyle and constipation is fairly well documented. For instance, the National Health and Nutrition Examination Survey published in 1989 found a twofold increased risk of constipation associated with low physical activity. In the famous ongoing Harvard Nurses' Health Study, which monitors the risk factors of chronic disease in thousands of women, physical activity two to six times per week was shown to lower the risk of constipation by more than a third.

Move against Gallstones

Gallbladder disease is often treated with surgery. Yet the nutritional and lifestyle risk factors of this disease are not well understood. Research suggests that a sedentary lifestyle along with a diet rich in animal fats and refined sugars and deficient in vegetable fats and fibers can promote gallstone formation. That was the main conclusion drawn from a 1999 Italian study comparing the lifestyle of 100 patients with newly diagnosed gallstones and 290 randomly selected individuals without the disease.

A Harvard study the year before concluded that 34 percent of symptomatic gallstone cases in men could be prevented by increasing their physical activity to 30 minutes daily five times a week. Among the other findings: men who watched television more than forty hours per week had a higher risk of painful gallstones than men who watched less than six hours.

The evidence suggests that physical activity also helps lower the amount of cholesterol in the biliary tract, a factor that could help prevent gallstones.

Move for a Healthier Liver

People don't appreciate the liver, the body's chief chemical factory. The liver masterminds the processing and utilization of the carbohydrates, fats, and proteins that you eat. It also removes toxic substances that have accumulated in the body. When its complex system goes wrong, you can suffer in many ways.

Today there is a growing epidemic called *fatty liver disease*. It ranges from a little bit of fat in the liver, which may not affect you at all, to something more serious called NASH—*nonalcoholic steatohepatosis*. In its more serious form, excess fat produces a high tide of inflammatory substances that irritate and even kill liver cells. These harmful agents also affect the cardiovascular system, the brain, and the liver. The medical community has tended to lump these things together as a benign kind of liver disease. We look at it differently.

NASH has a 60 percent five-year survival rate. That's chronic liver failure. When fat cells move into the liver or any other tissue, they are not just benign cells moving in next door. Fat cells are active players. They churn out inflammatory molecules. Those molecules not only get into the whole system, but they interfere with the normal cells around them, disturbing routine cellular functions. Inside the liver, they cause damage to an organ you definitely want operating as efficiently as possible.

Our bodies have evolved to store excess energy (such as fat) wherever they can, including in the liver, so that when lean times come and we have no access to food, our bodies can readily convert the stored fat to energy. The problem is that over the last half-century or so, we have put ourselves in a constant storage mode even though we never lack access to food. It's a survival function of the body, but it hurts us if we are inactive and not burning off the energy stores. Putting it in banking terms, the liver constantly gets the deposits but there are no withdrawals. So it gets fat.

CLOCK YOUR PROGRESS

Here's how quickly physical activity can benefit your digestive health and elimination:

- Within two weeks: less heartburn, better bowel function, and often relief of constipation.
- Long term: reduces risk of GI tract cancers, including pancreatic, liver, and colon cancers; reduces risk of diverticulosis and diverticulitis.

As you pack away extra fat in the liver, liver enzymes start to rise. That's a red flag indicating the liver isn't happy with what's going on. We routinely see from imaging studies and enzyme results that consistent physical activity reverses this situation. A desirable withdrawal of stored fat takes place. As the withdrawals continue, liver operations improve.

We have published studies showing that the more physically active you are, the less liver fat you have, no matter what your overall weight is. If you take two people at the same weight, the person who is more physically active will have less liver fat.

The emphasis among physicians and among researchers is always on weight. You're too fat, and therefore you have fat in your liver. There is never any focus on physical activity.

We find a strong connection here to visceral adiposity—the deep-down belly fat that's a by-product of sedentary living. If you look at the *hepatoportal* circulation—that is, the blood circulating through your gut area— all roads lead to the liver. The blood passes directly through the liver. Visceral fat pumps out a steady stream of inflammatory substances and fatty molecules and they flow right down the expressway to the liver.

Visceral fat goes hand in hand with liver fat. In fact, it is the strongest predictor of liver fat. Physical activity reduces visceral adiposity, which subsequently reduces liver fat.

Move to Reduce Pain

Sally was a seventy-six-year-old retired accountant when she responded to one of our radio advertisements seeking sedentary individuals to participate in a walking study. She was a prime subject for our study. She had never exercised in her life. She was overweight with poor mobility and pain in her legs, and she needed a cane for support when she walked. She always seemed to have a cold or some physical ailment. The thought of exercise scared her. She was fearful it would be too much for her, that she might fall and injure herself. Walking up one flight of stairs, or walking on a flat surface longer than a few minutes at a time required that she stop and take a five- to ten-minute breather.

After a couple of months into the study she was a transformed woman. She was walking for up to 20 minutes a day several or more times a week and was "amazed" that she could now sustain physical activity. Moreover, she didn't need a cane anymore, and her pain level had decreased considerably.

"I never realized I was in such pathetic shape until I saw the difference that a little bit of exercise can do," she told us.

You know the old saying, "That's the way the cookie crumbles." Well, guess what? If you are sedentary, you become a crumbling cookie. Your muscles, ligaments, and tendons weaken and your body basically crumbles, creating imbalances, misalignments, and a domino effect of irregular forces throughout the musculoskeletal system. Aches, pains, and arthritis result.

Over time, sedentary individuals lose their functional muscle mass, a process of slow deterioration due to disuse. The use-it-or-lose-it principle is unmercifully at work here. As you slowly crumble away, your skeletal frame has a harder time being held erect by muscles that are smaller and weaker. The risk of overuse injury increases, and you start developing all the "itises" associated with tendons and ligaments. Sedentary patients frequently complain of painful tendonitis and bursitis. They often tell us they are reluctant to pursue physical activity out of fear they will hurt more and make things worse. Although some people sincerely believe this, most know better. To us, it's a justification for doing nothing. Rest assured that if you do nothing, you will hurt more and make things worse in the long run.

Sedentary patients often tell us they feel they are getting stiffer and their joints are more achy. They blame age. It's not age. It's the muscles supporting the joints that are getting weaker. And the joints function less efficiently as a result.

In our quality-of-life patient survey, 34 percent of sedentary, low-fitness patients said they had significant chronic muscle or joint pain. For moderately fit patients, 29 percent responded affirmatively. In the high-fitness

CLOCK YOUR PROGRESS

Here's how quickly physical activity can help with muscular and joint pain problems:

- Within weeks: pain reduction, better joint mobility, better range of motion.
- Months to years: a process of improving joint health from strengthened muscles, ligaments, and tendons, which reduces the risk of degenerative joint disease, including osteoarthritis.

category, only 23.5 percent reported pain, almost a third fewer patients than in the low-fitness group.

People commonly think that if you exercise, you will wear out your joints. Just the opposite is true. Our clinical experience over the years clearly shows that the more physically active you are, the lower your risk of developing arthritis is. The medical literature confirms our observations.

Even a modest physical activity routine—like our Plan A described in part two—starts to quickly rebuild and strengthen the soft-tissue structures that support the skeleton and joints.

Physical activity boosts blood flow, an overlooked element for healthy joints. Improved blood flow means you can better supply nutrients to the ends of the bone tissue adjacent to working joints. One common but little-known hip problem is called *avascular necrosis* of the head of the femur, meaning not enough blood is reaching the upper end of the thigh bone. This vulnerable area becomes even more threatened when certain steroidal anti-inflammatory medications, called *glucocorticoids*, are used in high doses or for long periods of time. Repetitive injuries and a sedentary lifestyle also raise the risk. Patients often need hip replacements because the blood supply is poor.

Hip pain caused by this condition indicates the joint is already in bad shape. Patients will usually get the diagnosis from an orthopedic surgeon, and in this case, the treatment is not physical activity. You'll need to treat the pain and at some point have a hip replacement. Young people can also suffer from this condition.

Often we get people back into activity with a temporary anti-inflammatory prescription—to ease existing pain—and then wean them off the medication as their functional status improves. By themselves, all the painkillers in the world won't heal a thing or strengthen the body.

The best prescription is to carefully recondition weak and sore tissue in a way that doesn't irritate it. For instance, avoid impact exercises or any extreme, intense activity that will exacerbate joint soreness. As for running, it doesn't put people at greater risk for joint pain unless they run far—sixty, seventy, or eighty miles a week—in which case they increase their risk slightly. For the most part, physical activity promotes healthy joints and reduces the risk of arthritis.

To us doctors, it is so gratifying to observe patients slowly and subtly improving over time after they start on a physical activity program. When patients revisit us, we show them their medical history forms from the year before. When we point out their comments about joint or muscle pain the year before, they will often say, "Oh, yes, I forgot all about that. The pain isn't there as much," or sometimes, "Oh that pain, well, it went away and I forgot all about it."

Move against Lower Back Pain

In our clinical approach to back pain, we find that many cases tend to be resolved over time when treatment includes a regular activity program. It doesn't happen in days or weeks. It happens over months.

Among the many causes of back pain, a sedentary lifestyle is often overlooked. In our survey of patient quality-of-life issues, we found that 45 percent of low-fitness individuals indicated they had had a significant lower back pain problem. Among moderately fit individuals, the incidence was 41.5 percent. The highly fit folks had the lowest incidence: 35 percent. For sure, weaker back muscles caused by physical inactivity give you less protection against the common causes of back pain.

Professionals in the field of rehabilitation medicine have been saying for years that physical fitness and aerobic conditioning can help both to reduce and prevent the occurrence of lower back pain. Some have pointed out in the medical literature that the passive nature of most treatment methods is a "major obstacle" to recovery. Prolonged bed rest, for instance, promotes a loss of bone and muscle mass, whereas proper physical movement enhances disk nutrition and ligament and tendon strength.

Most people assume that we develop back pain and lose height because of the spinal vertebrae settling on top of each other. That happens only minimally. The real reason is that as we age the shoulders roll forward, the head tilts forward, and the whole upper body sags forward. Arthritic changes occur in the spine to some extent in most people, but you want to try to keep the spine as erect as possible by consciously keeping the shoulders back. The perennial command of the drill sergeant is right on: "Chest out, shoulders back, stomach in." Try to apply it consciously in your daily activities. Thus, if arthritis occurs, it happens more in a straight line than in an unsightly curve.

Think of the spine as a tower. Think of the *paraspinus* muscles—the muscles running up and down along the spine—and the abdominal muscles as the guide wires. If the guide wires are strong, the tower remains optimally erect. If the guide wires are weak because of a sedentary lifestyle, the tower can't support the top floor—in this case your 10-pound head. You'll get the sag, and with it, the neck pain and the back pain. The muscles aren't strong enough to hold things up. They tire faster. The neck, shoulders, and back tighten up.

Should you have massage therapy for the neck and shoulder? Sure, that will help you. But you really need to strengthen the core muscles of your belly and back so you can hold yourself in a more correct posture.

But for a start, any type of low-impact general fitness program works these muscles. Walking is as good an activity as any. While you don't directly work these muscles with walking, you engage them. You start retoning them. And you will feel better.

Move to Combat Fibromyalgia

Fibromyalgia is somewhat of a wastebasket diagnosis. It's often a handy label when physicians can't figure out the real problem. Many people who receive the diagnosis probably don't really have the condition. Fibromyalgia involves chronic musculoskeletal pain in association with multiple tender points on the body, muscle stiffness, fatigue, headaches, and sleep disturbances. This is really a condition of exclusion. You have to first exclude underlying rheumatologic, orthopedic, metabolic, and psychological problems such as depression. Making an accurate diagnosis is difficult because symptoms vary so much from person to person and the complaints are fairly generalized and overlapping.

Patients' complaints usually sound like this:

- "I ache all over."
- "I hurt like I never hurt before."
- "I'm tired and get easily fatigued."

We've seen many people at the clinic with a diagnosis of fibromyalgia, but very few of them have had the appropriate workup from their family doctors to confirm it medically. Often we find problems such as occupational stress, depression, a vertebral disk problem, or the effects of midlife hormonal changes.

If indeed you have fibromyalgia, we recommend regular, light physical activity. You don't want to compromise muscle tone and metabolic efficiency and raise the risk of many of the health problems described in this book caused by inactivity. At the same time, activity intensity must be kept low to avoid aggravating the body.

In general, our fibromyalgia prescription is to walk five times a week for 10 minutes initially, eventually increasing the time so that a mile is covered in 20 minutes. Patients tell us they start feeling better with that kind of simple approach.

A British study confirmed our observations about the benefits of activity as a treatment for fibromyalgia. In the study, rheumatologists randomly divided 136 fibromyalgia patients into two experimental groups. One group was assigned light physical activity, and the other group was assigned to do relaxation techniques along with some stretching. At the end of three months, the participants filled out questionnaires rating their health status. Significantly more of them in the exercise group rated themselves as much better or very much better, and reported greater reductions in tender point intensity. Some of the benefits lasted an entire year. The exercise program consisted of mostly walking on treadmills or cycling on stationary bikes. At the start, participants came for two sessions per week that lasted about 6 minutes. They were encouraged to increase the time gradually and as tolerated. By twelve weeks they were doing 25 minutes at an intensity that made them sweat slightly while still being able to converse comfortably in complete sentences. The doctors heading the study concluded that individualized aerobic exercise is a "simple, cheap, effective" treatment for fibromyalgia.

Move for Headache Relief

Headaches run the gamut from background nuisance to severe, sidelining blockbusters. Nearly thirty million Americans, for instance, suffer

CLOCK YOUR PROGRESS
How fast can physical activity impact a headache problem? Within months, many patients report improvements.

from migraine headaches, one of the more severe types. Women are three times more likely than men to experience migraines. Certainly, medications can help with acute episodes as well as with prevention; however, one tool that is grossly underutilized for preventing headaches is physical activity.

In 2006 Dr. Mitchell, in his capacity as health columnist for *USA Weekend*, interviewed Merle Diamond, M.D., associate director of the famous Diamond Headache Clinic in Chicago. She said that at her clinic, physical activity is a standard part of the therapy program to reduce the incidence of headaches.

The same is also true of headache treatment at the Cooper Clinic. We have found that sedentary patients who suffer from headaches get gradual relief to varying degrees when they sustain a program of physical activity.

In our quality-of-life survey, we asked patients whether they suffered from frequent headaches. Of the sedentary, low-fitness group, nearly 17 percent answered yes. In the moderate-fitness category, 15 percent said yes. For the highly fit folks, the response was 12 percent.

Unlike many other health associations, the link between headaches and physical activity has not been widely researched. Findings do suggest, however, that physically active people tend to be less bothered by headaches.

Move to Live Better Longer

Hal, seventy-one, is a retired business executive with one house in Florida and another in Dallas. At 245 pounds, he's far too heavy for his 5-foot-10-inch frame. We can always tell whether he has been active or not when he comes in for routine checkups. Most of the time he stays active by walking outdoors for up to 30 minutes a day. That's his preference. His weight doesn't fluctuate much, however, whether he's active or not. What fluctuates are his medical test results.

With all the hurricanes that hit Florida in 2004 and 2005, he wasn't able to be as active as usual. At one point, he had to evacuate his house. When he came for checkups after periods of weather-induced inactivity, his medical test numbers had deteriorated. They typically improve when he stays active.

Hal will never get skinny, but he says that when he stays active he feels the best.

Hal is a typical example of someone who benefits from physical activity, even though he is too heavy and is likely to stay that way as long as he continues to overeat and to drink excessively, as is his habit. By treadmill standards, he is a fit man. Far too heavy, but fit.

The benefits for Hal and for other seniors, regardless of weight, are truly precious. Physical activity prevents, minimizes, and reverses the strength, flexibility, and functional slowdown that comes with aging— even for sedentary people who become active at an advanced age. It can preserve independent living longer into old age.

The potential dividends for the elderly were highlighted in a 2004 *Washington Post* article by Rob Stein titled, "It's Never Too Late to Be Healthy, Studies Show." Stein showcased four new studies concluding that a healthy lifestyle—including physical activity—produces dramatic benefits for aging bodies and minds.

In an editorial accompanying one of the studies in the *Journal of the American Medical Association*, Meir J. Stampfer of the Harvard School of Public Health remarked that "a lot of times older people get the idea that, 'What's done is done. It's too late for me.'" The research, he pointed out, shows that "it's not too late to have a big influence."

As an example, take the following 2006 experiment with sedentary Florida seniors, with an average age of eighty-three and a half years. In this study, Robert Simons of the Bonsai Spa and Wellness Clinic in Largo and Ross Andel of the University of South Florida's School of Aging Studies explored the effects of sixteen weeks of supervised resistance training and walking exercise on various measures of functional and cardiovascular fitness.

Forty-five women and nineteen men participated, all residents of an independent living facility. They were split into several groups: one involved in self-paced walking, a second in a simple resistance (strength) training program, and a third that served as a comparison group with no changes. The two active groups engaged in exercise just twice a week.

All participants were tested at the start of the trial and then again at the conclusion. Compared to the nonactive group, the walkers and strength trainers made significant gains in functional fitness. The most substantial improvements in the walking group were in upper- and lower-body strength, coordination, and hip flexibility. The strength-training group improved most in upper- and lower-body strength and coordination as well, but also in agility and balance.

Studies like this are important because adults more than eighty years old are the fastest-growing segment of the population, and they are more prone to a sedentary lifestyle than younger people. The research clearly shows that previously sedentary adults at an advanced age have much quality of life to gain just by adding a bit of physical activity to their daily routines.

PART TWO

The Cooper Center Move Yourself Programs

4

Choose the Right Program for You

We are under exercised as a nation. We look instead of play. We ride instead of walk. Our growing softness, our increasing lack of physical fitness, is a menace to our security.

—John F. Kennedy

We have tossed you a lot of good reasons to get moving. Hopefully, we have convinced you of how much you stand to gain in health and quality of life. We'll assume we have made our case and that you are ready to roll now and won't put it off until your next New Year's resolutions.

Before proceeding, take a minute to note the personal reasons you're choosing to become physically active. What's in it for you?

Clinical health psychologist Jay Ashmore, Ph.D., director of the weight-loss program at our center, asks all participants that question before they start. These are some of the typical responses he receives:

- "My father had a heart attack in his forties. I don't want to die young."
- "I want to be around when my kids grow up and have kids of their own."
- "I feel lousy. I want to feel better."
- "I look bad."
- "I'm too fat."
- "I want to find a significant other."

When people tell him they have young kids and want to be around for the grandkids, Ashmore reminds them about the importance of being good fitness and nutrition role models. "Kids relate more to what you do than to what you say," he tells them.

Whatever your reasons for getting active, write them on a piece of paper and keep it in this book so you can refer back to it later. Also write down any health issues or symptoms that you would like to see improved by physical activity. At the end of every month, as you sustain a physical activity program, record your progress and improvements.

What Plan Is Right for You?

Our physical activity prescription includes three plans, so let's make sure you start with the plan that fits you best. Use the chart below for guidance.

| | Where You Are Now | | |
Your Goal	Sedentary	Partially Active	Active
Better Health	Plan A	Increase the number of days you are active. Use Plan A concepts to achieve that goal.	Plan B
Better Health + Fitness	Become consistent with Plan A, then proceed very slowly with Plan B.	Move up to Plan B once you are consistently active.	Plan B
Better Health + Fitness + Waist Removal and Weight Loss	Become consistent with Plan A, and then with Plan B. Only then proceed to Plan C.	Advance from Plan B to Plan C.	Plan C

Likely, you fit into the Plan A category, meaning you are sedentary according to the physical activity quiz and step counter test you took in chapter 1. Please don't fool yourself. You need to know how fit—or unfit—you are today, not how active you were ten or twenty years ago. Plan A will first and foremost improve your health. It is our gentle start-up program that practically anybody can follow. It eases you into physical activity in a safe, comfortable, and effective way. Plan A generates enough fitness to improve your health and quality of life, and to neutralize some of the visceral fat you may have acquired over the years. Remember: the greatest benefits come from raising yourself up a notch from low-fitness status to moderate fitness—going from doing nothing to doing something, even if it's just a minimum amount of activity.

If you are partially active, perhaps a weekend warrior, or you go to the gym once or twice a week, you can probably start with Plan B. If you have any doubts, start with Plan A. It's a lot of fun anyway, even if you are an active person. Higher levels of fitness call for an expanded program of aerobic activity, such as walking, jogging, cycling, or swimming, along with some strength training and stretching exercises. Don't try Plan B if you are presently sedentary.

If your ultimate goal is major trimming of visceral fat and overall body weight, eventually you'll need to move up to Plan C. We call it our waist-removal program. But don't start there if you are sedentary. It's a plan requiring physical activity at a much greater intensity and frequency than either of the other plans.

Be Smart, Be Safe

No matter which plan you follow, please be prudent. Speak to your doctor first and get clearance, especially if you have any chronic medical condition and you intend to ramp up your activity level considerably. We recommend that anyone over forty have a checkup before beginning a physical activity program. Even if you are already active and want to go to a higher level of fitness, check with your doctor.

Your doctor's clearance is particularly critical if you have a history of heart trouble, such as irregular rhythms, or have had an actual heart attack. Chest pain is a common sign of heart disease. If you have it, consult with your physician before you attempt any program of physical activity.

Check your doctor if you feel faint or dizzy when you exercise. Faintness or dizziness can be related to many things, such as illness, heat, or dehydration. It could also be related to a weak heart.

If you have any bone or joint condition (for instance, problems with your knees, hips, or back) ask your doctor which form of activity is the safest and most effective for you.

If you have been inactive for many years, be very careful when starting out. If you are too aggressive, you can injure yourself. Remember, you do not have the same body you had twenty years ago. Don't go crazy and think you are a kid again.

The story of Chad, one of our patients for many years, is a tragic example of what not to do. He was an ex-Marine, a driven, type A person, busy at work but not exercising. He had a history of high blood pressure.

After he hit fifty, his world seemed to cave in. He lost a daughter in a car accident, he was laid off from his job, and his wife filed for divorce. The stress was overwhelming and his blood pressure worsened.

When we saw him last, however, he had landed a new job, his life had settled down a bit, and he had started exercising again—hard. Working out became his feel-good outlet in life. He was pushing himself. He dropped an extra 15 to 20 pounds.

His gung-ho military spirit had kicked in. If walking was good, running was better. And he was running hard.

But there was danger in his constant pushing. Chad was fifty-nine, with high blood pressure and some plaque building up in his coronary arteries. We warned him. Our very last words to him went something like this:

"It's great that you are taking care of yourself now. But you are not twenty anymore. There is a difference between exercise for performance and activity for health. You are overdoing it. Be careful."

"Got you," he said. "Got you."

But apparently he didn't get it. In November 2005, on a business trip, he keeled over coming out of the fitness center in his hotel. He suffered a fatal heart attack.

The intensity of his workouts could have caused an unstable coronary plaque to rupture from an excess of sheer force—the tangential pressure of flowing blood on arterial walls. Instead of *training* his heart, he may have been *straining* his heart.

As we get older, we often think of ourselves as still being twenty. More often than not, it's a guy thing. Machismo. More common than Chad's story is the damage we see people do to themselves by not respecting their age or condition. One of our patients, not a regular exerciser, suffered a significant hamstring pull when he decided to challenge a friend to a hundred-yard dash during a fund-raising rally at their children's school. The first five steps of the sprint were easy, but six steps into the race he was reminded of his age and condition. He caused a tear in his rear end and leg and needed months to recover from it. As Clint Eastwood said at the end of the 1973 movie classic *Magnum Force*, "A man's got to know his limitations."

We see many men—and women—at our clinic who once played sports in high school and college, then got married, launched their careers, and stopped exercising. Their personal point of reference for activity is exercise for *performance*. We try to persuade them to shift their thinking now that they are older—away from activity for *performance* to activity for *health*. We try to get them away from the "no pain, no gain" attitude, and the idea that if you don't go out there and play singles tennis for a couple of hours you haven't done anything. This is a very common and self-defeating mind-set. They may tell us they don't have the time to exercise the way they used to. We tell them they don't need to. They just need to exercise a little. Some exercise is better than none at all.

It's Never Too Late

Use it or lose it.

—Tennis great Jimmy Connors

We know from our patients and study participants that it is never too late to start a physical activity routine. We have witnessed remarkable improvements among individuals sixty-five and even much older who have had heart attacks or some chronic illness.

Our data show that regardless of advanced age, gender, or previous health, the benefits are right there waiting for you to take possession. If you are sedentary and elderly, you just need to get moving—even minimally—to ignite the process. Start with Plan A, and then if you wish, very slowly and very, very gently, as your individual condition allows, you can add some elements of light strength training and flexibility described in Plan B.

Be sure to check with your physician before you get started. And if you can afford it, work with a qualified trainer who can assist you personally and take any physical limitations into consideration. If you can't afford a one-on-one trainer, encourage several activity-minded friends to participate with you and collectively hire the trainer. It's more fun exercising in a group, anyway.

The Busy-Active Conundrum

"I am very busy and active all day."

That's a common response we hear from participants in our many studies with sedentary populations, from people of all ages, socioeconomic levels, and races. It never ceases to amaze us just how sedentary many of these people are, often without being aware of it. They believe they are active because they are busy throughout the day and are tired at the end of the day. They work at jobs or take care of children, have social lives, and go through the stresses of everyday life. Their routines fatigue them. They don't feel like going to a gym or taking a walk.

"I'm too tired," or, "I just don't have time," they will tell us. If health is a concern, many say they will deal with it later on in life. Right now, they are too busy dealing with their present concerns. It's hard for them to adopt physical activity as a prevention strategy for something that may happen in the future.

We find that sedentary folks usually have some health or mood problems, and when they come to the center for initial interviews, many become out of breath just by walking the hundred feet from the parking lot into our building. Most arrive breathing hard at our exercise lab after walking one short flight of stairs from the reception desk.

Our interviews uncover some interesting subthemes. For instance, the attitude factor. With older individuals (sixty and over), particularly women, we run into a generational attitude toward activity. Many older women have simply never been physically active. Exercise wasn't encouraged when they were younger. They never participated in sports or physical activity for body image. It is practically a foreign concept to them.

Among younger people, from age thirty to the early fifties, the men often say the problem is their work schedule. They jumped on the corporate train and never got off.

For women it's often work, too, as well as kids and family. "I've been so busy taking care of everybody else that I've had no time to take care of myself," they will say.

The Challenge for Moms

We'll sometimes encounter mothers who say they are so busy running around that they have no time for exercise, and besides, they say they get plenty of physical activity just chasing after the kids. Generally, mothers indeed get some physical activity, but not as much as they think. Yes, they might carry a child to the car and then from the car to the shopping cart. But the concept that mothering involves a lot of physical activity is not supported by the evidence. Mothers are just as sedentary as everyone else.

In a presentation at a 1999 scientific meeting of the American Heart Association, a University of Minnesota researcher found that parenthood resulted in less leisure-time physical activity for women, but not for men. That comes as no surprise, since women are frequently more involved in caring for kids, said Kathryn Schmitz. Because of that, women need special time or programs that allow them to exercise with their children present. The biggest drop for moms in physical activity occurs with the first child, and activity doesn't pick up with additional children. Schmitz's conclusions were based on data from questionnaires completed by 3,274 black and white participants over a ten-year period.

Granted, mothers may be exhausted at day's end, but the fatigue often comes from lack of sleep or the kids driving them nuts, not from physical activity per se.

We acknowledge that women tend to be the caretakers of the family. They take care of husbands, kids, the house, and with only so much time in the day, they may become lax about taking care of themselves. Many, of course, also work outside of the home, leaving them with even less extra time.

Women are nurturers, generally programmed to think of others first. For some, the thought of taking time out of the day to exercise for their own well-being borders on the selfish. But here's the reality and the challenge: in order to take good care of others you have to take care of yourself, because if your health breaks down, you won't be able to take care of anyone else.

So although they are busy, many women are not physically active at a beneficial level. But exercising to that level is not as difficult as they may think. They carpool kids, shop, buy groceries, do laundry, and often eat on the run. While doing all that, they have plenty of opportunities to add bits of activity with very little effort. In the pages ahead, we'll describe how to do just that.

Move Yourself Plan A

Getting Active— the Easy, Fun Way

If you are sedentary, and if the thought of vigorous exercise turns you off, you have come to the right place. Plan A stands for Active, and it eases you into physical activity in a safe, comfortable, effective, easy, and fun way. With Plan A you will move yourself from low fitness to moderate fitness, and reap the greatest health benefits in the process.

Plan A is doable for everyone. You take it at your own pace, counting your steps and gradually learning how to fit physical activity into your schedule. You will also learn to be mindful of your eating habits, and to decide where to make healthier choices.

Later you may want to move on to Plan B, but even if you just stick with Plan A, you will be giving yourself a considerable health advantage.

5

Step Counting and Logging: Your Keys to Success

A journey of a thousand miles begins with a single step.
—Confucius

Hopefully, we've motivated you to get up and get moving, but we realize that if you are sedentary, you may not know where to begin. That's why we've created four success keys to ease the start of your physical activity regimen. According to Confucius, you only need one step to get started. So, with four steps, you're ahead of the game!

Success Key 1: Buy a Step Counter

Your master key to jump-starting the Plan A physical activity program is to get yourself a step counter. It's the only piece of equipment you'll need.

For us doctors, it is always difficult to get patients to follow our physical activity recommendations. In our experience, the step counter usually eliminates the compliance problem, because patients have so much fun using it. A step counter measures your physical activity by counting the number of steps you take. You clip the device onto your belt or waistband. You'll be amazed at how much this device motivates physical activity.

Steve Blair, our former director of research, introduced the step counter in the United States in 1992 after traveling to Japan to visit an exercise physiology professor who had begun using it there. A Japanese company making step counters donated two hundred and fifty devices to Blair, and that enabled our center to get the first study going.

"The step counter is like any intervention—pills or otherwise—and not every one thing works for everybody," he says. "But people really like using this gadget. We've put it to the test in many studies. It can be a great boost to getting people into physical activity and keeping them there."

As we mentioned earlier, you can purchase a step counter at most sporting goods stores or you can order one from our center for around $20. We have also produced a booklet called *Steps to Better Health* ($6.95) to help maximize your step counter use. These items are available at the Cooper Clinic store. (See page 17 for contact information.)

We have hundreds of step counters in action every day in our research to identify sedentary people and to track physical activity during exercise studies. We also use these devices very successfully in weight-management studies, and every person who enters a weight loss program at our center gets one. This is how we log our patients' physical activity. We have access to thousand-dollar accelerometers, very high-tech equipment that you wear on your belt, to track physical activity. We have found, however, that the inexpensive step counters are just as good and are amazingly accurate.

Step counter or pedometer—is there a difference? You can sometimes find both at sporting goods stores. A step counter simply registers steps. Pedometers do the same but some offer additional features, such as converting steps to an estimated distance covered by using your average stride length. Some models convert steps to calories via a preprogrammed formula, but they don't take into account age, gender, or intensity of activity. They give a rough calorie estimate. In any case, either a step counter or a pedometer monitors your steps.

Step counters are quite easy to use, but here are a few guidelines to help you get started.

To wear the step counter correctly, attach it securely to your belt or waistband. Position it on a straight line above your knee, unless the directions that came with the device say otherwise. If you don't attach the step counter correctly, it won't count steps accurately and you risk losing it. If you wear a dress or other clothing that does not have a waistband, attach the device to the waistband of your undergarment, or some kind of elastic that you wear over or under your clothes.

Studies have found that the step counter gives an accurate count, but you should test it to make sure.

- Set the device to zero, and attach it to your belt or waistband.
- Take 50 steps. Count the steps as you move. Each individual foot forward is one step.
- Stop and check your step counter. Is the total within 5 steps of 50? If so, your device passes the accuracy test and you can expect to use it with good effect to accurately log your steps. If the total is out of the accuracy range, set the counter to zero again and make sure you attach the device correctly.
- Try the 50-step test again. If the number is still off, reposition the device further toward the hip. Test it again. If it's still off, there may be a battery problem. You may need to contact the manufacturer or supplier for help. Step counters contain a pendulum or level arm that responds to the motion of the hip. Each person's body structure is somewhat different, so the most accurate positioning of the counter may vary. You may need a few tries to find the best spot to attach it.

The step counter provides you with "real-time" data. Get in the habit of wearing it daily. At the end of the day leave it in a place where you can find it and slip it right on the next morning. That could be on your bedside table, next to your keys, or on top of the dresser—just someplace where you won't miss it.

Success Key 2:
Log Your Activity

We highly recommend that you use physical activity logs to track your activity, especially in the beginning. Activity logging is a simple but highly effective way to figure out where your time goes and what are the best opportunities for slipping physical activity into your daily routine. It's a kind of time-and-motion diary. We recommend the practice for three reasons: (1) it gets people to realize how really sedentary they are in a concrete, quantitative way; (2) it enables them to readily see opportunities in daily life where they can include physical activity; and (3) it's a powerful key to making lasting changes.

Okay, it does involve a small bit of personal paperwork, but nothing tedious. We've tried to make it easier by putting together some forms for you. You'll find them—both samples and blank forms—at the end of the chapter. Before filling out any of the blank forms, make copies so that you can use them as often as you want. We suggest you fill out a new form every day.

Take a look at the sample activity log on page 122. At our center, both patients and study participants fill out a form like this and use it as activity management guides. The log is where you'll start putting your step counter to work. By recording your steps, you can readily monitor your progress and see how you are advancing toward your goal.

Following the sample log you will find a blank log for your personal use. Use this form to record your daily activities for each of the time slots indicated. Some people prefer to create their own logs on the computer, daily planner, or calendar. Choose whichever way works for you.

Other helpful tips for completing your personal activity log:

- Keep your log with you and write things down as you go.
- At the end of each day, determine the total number of minutes you spent being physically active.

Success Key 3: Set Your Target

The Old Order Amish live pretty much as they did a hundred years ago. They don't drive automobiles. They don't use electrical appliances or other modern conveniences. Labor-intensive farming is still the preferred occupation. In 2004 researchers at the University of Tennessee studied 98 men and women—ages eighteen to seventy-five—in a Canadian Amish community, monitoring physical activity and adiposity. For a week, the study participants wore step counters and filled out a log sheet recording their activities and steps on a daily basis.

Their average steps per day were 18,425 for men and 14,196 for women. The men achieved those numbers from ten hours of vigorous physical activity, forty-three hours of moderate activity, and twelve hours of walking each week. Practically the only time they sat down was when they ate. They were living a whole lot more like our great-grandparents did. They ate a pre–World War II diet, consuming generous servings of bacon, eggs, and apple pie, but their incidence of obesity was only 4 percent as compared to 20 to 25 percent in the overall U.S. population.

The Amish way of life obviously involves a high level of physical activity. We don't expect Amish-type numbers from you. But how about 8,500 to 10,000 steps a day?

Steve Blair, who first brought step counters back from Japan in 1992, says that 10,000 steps a day was set as a healthy physical activity goal, based on the earlier Japanese experience using the device. Subsequent experience in the United States has confirmed that number as a great target for fitness and health. If you get there consistently, or even get close, consider yourself a success. That's the goal we tell our patients to aim for, and that's the goal you should set for yourself. Here's the simple strategy for getting there step by step.

Determine Your Starting Point

The first thing you need to do is find your activity starting point. That means your present activity level. You can determine that by wearing your step counter for three entire days (two weekdays and one weekend day). Wear it from the time you get out of bed in the morning until you go to bed at night. Obviously, don't take it into the shower or bathtub with you. And remember to clip it back on if you take it off when you visit the restroom.

To determine the most accurate starting point, follow your normal routine during the three days. Don't do any extra activity. Park your car where you always park it. Take the elevator to your office, and not the staircase, if that is your custom.

Make a copy of the blank Activity Starting Point Log (on page 124), and record the total number of steps you took each day. Remember to reset the counter to zero at the end of each day or first thing in the morning. At the end of the three days, add up the total steps you took and divide the sum by three. That will tell you how many steps on average you take each day. That's your starting point, your baseline. That's what you want to improve on.

Compare Yourself

We routinely put step counters on sedentary folks to measure their activity levels. The immediate feedback we usually get is: "I didn't realize just how inactive and sedentary I was."

We find that the folks who enter our weight management programs are averaging 2,000 to 3,000 steps a day. We have put step counters on hundreds of sedentary postmenopausal women and found that they average about 4,500 steps a day. Some people report as low as 1,500. Others with even smaller numbers are usually reluctant to report anything.

How do you compare?

To give you an idea of how little movement there may be in a "busy" day, here are a couple of typical daily logs, one for a middle-aged office manager, the other for a homemaker/mother:

OFFICE MANAGER LOG

Time	Activity	Steps
6 to 6:45 A.M.	Wake-up, shower/dress, breakfast	400
6:45 A.M.	Drive to work	100
7 to 9:30 A.M.	Meetings, phone calls, e-mails	300
9:30 to 10 A.M.	Coffee, social rounds, discussion	400
10 A.M. to Noon	Meeting, phone calls, e-mails	300
Noon to 1:15 P.M.	Walk to car, drive to lunch, lunch	250
1:15 to 6 P.M.	Meeting, phone calls, e-mails	300
6 to 6:40 P.M.	Drive home	100
6:40 to 7:30 P.M.	Dinner	200
7:30 to 9:30 P.M.	Taking care of affairs at home	350
9:30 to 11 P.M.	Relaxing, TV	200
11 P.M. to 6 A.M.	Sleep	0

Total steps: 2,900

HOMEMAKER/MOM LOG

Time	Activity	Steps
6 to 6:30 A.M.	Wake up, wash up	50
6:30 to 7 A.M.	Make lunches, start laundry	250
7 to 7:45 A.M.	Make breakfast, feed kids	300
7:45 to 8 A.M.	Drive kids to school	150
8 to 11:30 A.M.	Pick up dry cleaning, buy groceries	350
11:30 A.M. to 12:30 P.M.	Lunch with friends	300
12:30 to 2:30 P.M.	Unload groceries, pay bills, more laundry	500
2:30 to 3:15 P.M.	Pick up kids	150
3:15 to 3:45 P.M.	Snacks, change clothes, get kids back in car	350
3:45 to 4:30 P.M.	Soccer practice and dance drop-off	200
5:15 to 5:30 P.M.	Pick up soccer kid	200
5:30 to 5:45 P.M.	Pick up dance kid	50
5:45 to 6:15 P.M.	Cook dinner	400
6:15 to 7 P.M.	Dinner	100
7 to 8:15 P.M.	Helping with homework	250
8:15 to 9 P.M.	Baths and bedtime for kids	250
9 to 9:45 P.M.	More laundry, finish cleaning kitchen	300
9:45 to 11 P.M.	Mom's time	100
11 P.M. to 6 A.M.	Sleep	0

Total steps: 4,250

Step Counter Encounters

Tedd Mitchell's Story

Like most doctors, I always considered myself busy and active at work. I'm up and down, and all around, seeing patients all day long. But until the day I clipped on a step counter before work, I didn't realize just how sedentary my job is, even with my busy schedule. I checked the step counter at noon, and I had taken only 500 steps over the course of four hours. I was floored. The number was totally unacceptable to me.

My little experiment prompted me to start getting up between patients to go to the lab to pick up medical test results rather than waiting for the results to be brought to me. Rather than calling upstairs for the result of a CAT scan, I walk up and check it out myself.

I'm a sports medicine physician, but until I put on that step counter, I was a prime example of deluding myself, like a whole lot of people do, about being active as well as busy on the job. For the record, I run a couple of miles every morning and go to the gym a few times a week. So I do get in my exercise. I practice what I preach. However, it took the step counter to open my eyes to the deceptively sedentary nature of my work.

Tim Church's Story

I have talked up the value of step counters for years, yet never really wore one, primarily because I run four or five days a week and, on the job, have always considered myself an active worker. I try to avoid e-mailing or calling colleagues who are within walking distance. I try to get up and go talk to people directly. I am always walking around the facility to peek in on studies in progress and monitor exercise testing.

One day I decided to see just how much activity I accumulated in my routine workday. I put on a step counter. I logged 2,900 steps—smack in the sedentary category. I thought it must be mistake, so I kept the step counter on for nearly two weeks. It was no mistake. I averaged around 2,900 steps during my workdays. I had no idea I was so sedentary, despite all my good intentions to be active. This was particularly disturbing to me since I try to obtain additional physical activity throughout my day at the office.

What I learned was that anybody who puts on a step counter is in for a real surprise. You'll see firsthand why we are a sedentary nation. The experience reinforced my belief that all of us must inject some purposeful activity into our daily schedule.

Martin Zucker's Story

I'm a writer. I work at home. My job is about as sedentary as it gets. My work commute entails going from one room to the next, and then sitting in front of the computer for hours. Nevertheless, I always believed myself to be an active person.

I'm not a runner, like Doctors Mitchell and Church, but I enjoy long brisk walks and going hiking whenever possible.

When I started working on this book, I put on a step counter. I was curious to see how active I really was. What a shocker! On the days that I didn't walk, I found that I was taking 2,000 or 3,000 steps a day. That's seriously sedentary.

Jolted into action by the step counter, I was inspired to start walking *every* day and going farther than before. I get away from the computer more often during workdays, and I take short walking breaks, around the block, or even in the garden—yanking some weeds along the way.

The step counter can be quite a contagious contraption. It's fun to use. I gave one to my wife, and it inspired her to take daily walks on those days she doesn't go to the gym. Our experience has been so positive that we give step counters to friends and family as birthday gifts.

Success Key 4: Increase Your Step Goal Week by Week

We want you to reach your step goal gradually, so that by the end of one month you are taking 2,000 steps more a day than at present. You can do that comfortably in weekly increments of 500 steps. Here's the simple plan:

- Week 1: Increase your present daily activity by 500 steps.
- Week 2: Add another 500 steps.

- Week 3: Add still another 500 steps.
- Week 4: Add still another 500 steps.

As an example, if your starting point is 3,500 steps daily, raise the level to 4,000 steps per day throughout the first week. For the second week, increase it by another 500, to 4,500 per day. For the third week, go up to 5,000 daily, and then to 5,500 for the fourth week. You'll quickly get caught up in the challenge. Use the Weekly Progress Log (page 125) to chart your progress week after week.

If you think you can increase your daily steps by more than 500, go for it. But keep your goal realistic so you'll make steady progress. Even if you feel energized, don't dramatically accelerate your progress. If you push yourself too much, you run the risk of muscle soreness or injury, especially if you have been inactive for a long period of time. Stick to the plan and it will stick with you. Remember, the tortoise won the race, not the hare. No need to hurry, just to be regular.

Check the step counter throughout the day to see if you are on target to meet your step goal. For instance, if you have logged about 2,000 steps before lunch and your goal is 6,000 for the day, you know you need to put in some extra time at lunch or in the afternoon to catch up. You will find that the step counter is such a great motivating and fun tool that after a while you will actually go out of your way to get in extra "mileage" to raise your total. Keep in mind that you can gain 450 to 500 steps just by walking briskly for 5 minutes.

The step counter can indicate those parts of the day when you are the most sedentary and need to make adjustments. It will tell you if you are more sedentary in the morning, in the afternoon, or in the evening. After a while you will get an intimate feeling for your activity patterns, something you were not aware of before. It's a great way to analyze a fundamental aspect of your lifestyle.

If you can collect the bulk of your activity minutes and steps in one shot every day, that's fine with us. But accumulating steps sprinkled throughout the day works as well. It's not easy to keep track of short spurts of activity, such as when you park your car farther away, take the stairs instead of the elevator, or reel off a brisk 7-minute walk to lunch. But by using the step counter, you can see your daily total growing. As the total rises, you'll get more and more inspired to keep moving. And as you feel better in the process, you'll never want to let up.

One thing that step counters can't do is to track non-weight-bearing activities such as swimming, biking, and water aerobics. If you become involved in these or any other activities the step counter can't record, just make a note about the specific activity and the minutes spent at it in your weekly activity log.

Strategies to Increase Your Steps

Your own physical activity log will give you the clues for where in your daily routine you can add steps. Here's a list of improvement ideas that we share with our patients and study participants:

At home

- Take your dog for a daily walk.
- Listen to an audio book or your favorite radio talk show or music while you walk.
- Wash your car by hand instead of taking it to the car wash.
- Get a push mower for your lawn. Rake your lawn.
- Walk to the corner or around the block or through your apartment complex whenever you check your mailbox.
- Get involved in active and fun recreational activities: hiking, ice skating, bike rides, gardening, bowling, dancing. Get your family involved as well.
- Actively play with your young kids instead of watching them. They will love your involvement.
- Walk around your house during TV commercials. You can log many hundreds of extra steps a day during the breaks. Put away the remote control and get up and change the channels on your TV.
- Walk as you talk on your cordless phone.
- Walk to a nearby store for items you can easily carry.

At the office

- Every hour or so, take a hundred steps around your office or building. Put some physical activity breaks (even 2- or 5-minute breaks) into your day timer. Program your computer to sound off when it's time for a break.

- Take the stairs instead of the elevator. Start with even one flight and challenge yourself to add a flight every week or two.
- Don't e-mail or call anybody within four hundred feet of you. Walk to that person and give them the message directly.
- If you take public transportation, get off a stop before yours, and walk the rest of the way. Do the same on the way home. If you drive to work, park farther away in the parking lot. Walk the ramps in the parking garage if it is not dangerous.
- Walk to and from lunch, if possible. Ten minutes there and back could add up to an extra thousand steps.
- Take the long way to the restroom. Use the stairs, if possible.

Tips for busy moms

- Walk the kids to school if that's feasible. Or if you drive them, after you drop the kids off, take a walk.
- During soccer practice or one of your kids' activities, get up and walk around the field, or around the building. Let your kid do his or her thing. Instead of sitting and watching all the time, you do your thing.
- If you have a toddler, use the stroller as an opportunity to infuse some regular walking activity into your daily routine. In a 2004 Australian study, researchers found that taking the baby out for a stroller walk significantly reduced postpartum depression and increased the fitness level of new moms.

Errands and shopping

- Park in the farthest space from the store or mall.
- Walk around the mall before you start shopping.

Traveling tips

- Walk around the airport while waiting for a flight, or around the station while waiting for a train or bus.
- Walk between terminals at the airport instead of riding the moving sidewalk.

- For added calorie burning, carry your briefcase and overnight bag instead of wheeling them behind you.

- Stay at a hotel within walking distance of your main business or tourist activities.

- Walk to nearby restaurants.

- Instead of going directly from afternoon meetings to happy hour or dinner, give yourself an active happy hour. Get in some walking.

After One Month—What's Next?

After a month of logging your physical activity, it's a good time to check your progress and health status.

How do you feel compared to how you felt before you started?

What benefits have you gotten?

Write down the improvements you have observed on the same piece of paper where you listed your health issues and physical activity goals before you started.

Activity Logs

For each four-hour block of time describe how you spend your time and calculate your number of steps using a step counter. Try to record your activities at least every one to two hours so you can be as accurate as possible. Record the total number of steps at the bottom of the sheet.

SAMPLE ACTIVITY LOG

Date: 07/27/07   **Day of Week:** Wednesday

Time Slot	Tasks/Activities	Physically Active? Yes No	Steps
Midnight to 4:00 A.M.		no	
4:01 to 8:00 A.M.	Shower, dress, breakfast Drive to work	yes yes	350 100
8:01 A.M. to Noon	Desk work Walk to and from car at lunch	yes yes	150 500
12:01 to 4:00 P.M.	Meetings Walk to and from vending machine	yes yes	250 100
4:01 to 8:00 P.M.	Walk to and from meetings Drive home Dinner	yes yes yes	250 100 150
8:01 P.M. to Midnight	Tidying up at home Relaxing, TV	yes no	350
			Total Steps 2300

YOUR ACTIVITY LOG

Date: **Day of Week:**

Time Slot	Tasks/Activities	Physically Active? Yes No	Steps
Midnight to 4:00 A.M.			
4:01 to 8:00 A.M.			
8:01 A.M. to Noon			
12:01 to 4:00 P.M.			
4:01 to 8:00 P.M.			
8:01 P.M. to Midnight			
			Total Steps

ACTIVITY STARTING POINT LOG

	Day and Date	Daily Steps
1		
2		
3		
Total (add the daily step counts)		
Average Daily Steps (divide the total steps by 3)		

Weekly Progress Log (Sample)

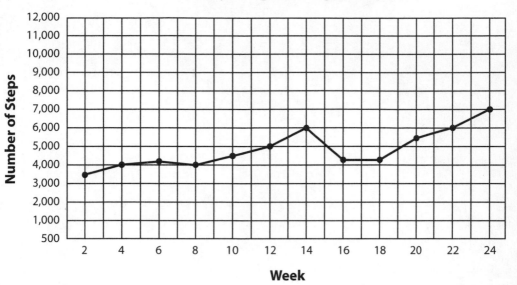

Your Weekly Progress Log

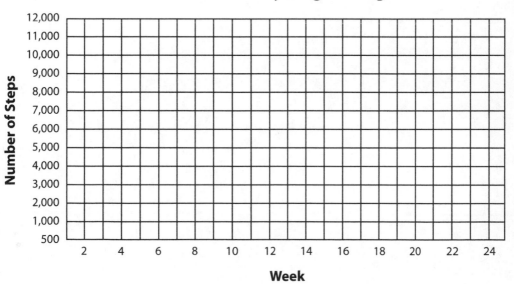

6

Keep Moving!
How to Stick with It

The road to success is dotted with many tempting parking places.
—Anonymous

K eep moving yourself, obviously! And keep reaping the health benefits of Plan A as you make physical activity a daily habit and priority. Keep recording your improvements.

Use the Weekly Progress Log to keep track of your daily steps over a six-month period. By following your steps week by week, you can see the big picture at a glance. You can see where you started and how far you've come along.

Don't worry if you fail to meet your quota each and every week. Have the intention to reach your target and then maintain it. Intention is all-important.

Common Excuses

As you push toward your long-term goal, you'll likely have times when you don't meet your daily goal. Don't worry. That happens to a lot a people. You run into obstacles, or events occur in your life that knock you temporarily off the path. Make sure the knock-offs are temporary. Remember that you need physical activity to stay healthy, so don't be sidetracked for long. It's what you do for the long haul that counts. If you find your activity level reverting back toward the sedentary, you will need to take some remedial action.

Here are some common obstacles—or excuses—for not being active, and some simple solutions:

"The weather's bad."

- Walk a nearby mall, the hallways of your office building, or the stairway at home or work.
- Vacuum the carpet. Clean your house aerobically, with lots of energy.

"I've got a house full of guests."

- Plan active events with them.
- Take a group walk while the food is in the oven or right after eating.

"It's hard to exercise because I'm traveling."

- Make sure when you travel that your feet do some traveling as well. If you are driving a long distance, stop occasionally and walk for 5 or 10 minutes.
- Use the hotel fitness center treadmill or ask about safe walking routes in the neighborhood. Walk the hotel stairways.

"I'm too tired."

- It's time to get up and move. Physical activity generates energy.
- Take a 10-minute walk. Once you get moving, you'll likely find it easy to keep moving.

"I'm lonely. I'm depressed."

- Walk your dog if you have one.
- Find a walking or physical activity partner, and give him or her permission to get on your case if you slack off. Talk in person, on the phone, or send an e-mail on a daily or weekly basis and let your partner know how much you have done and how you feel. If

you have a problem getting enough physical activity, brainstorm on how to find more opportunities during the day. Reporting to somebody who holds you accountable makes you more diligent and also helps overcome loneliness.

- Remind yourself that physical activity is a great antidote for depression. If you feel depressed, write down how you feel and then go out for a walk. Write down how you feel after you return. Follow this simple strategy when you feel down. Do it until you get to the point that when you start feeling depressed, you automatically get up and go out for a walk because you know from experience that you will feel better. Patients tell us frequently that when they come back from that little walk, they feel better about themselves and less inclined to reach for a fattening snack. Even our very depressed patients tell us that the activity uplifts and energizes them so much, they may go around the block not just once but two or three times.

"I'm bored."

- Spice up your physical activity routine. Buy someone you like a step counter (a very "fitting" birthday or holiday gift) and set up a friendly challenge. See who can log more steps by noon or by the end of designated days.

- Set up a friendly step count competition in your office or family. Create a prize for the winner.

- Once you get up to speed, benefit others with your growing level of fitness by participating in a charity run or walk event. It not how fast you do it, it's just about *doing* it.

"A loved one is hospitalized."

- If you have to take time out of your daily routine to be with a hospitalized family member or close friend, you can still do little things to take care of yourself. Park as far from the hospital entrance as possible. Take the stairs instead of the elevator. While waiting for a doctor or nurse, take a 5-minute walk up and down the stairs or hallway. Use any situation to look for creative physical activity opportunities.

"I forget to be active."

- Post reminders around your house or in your office.
- Write BE ACTIVE! in red ink every day on your calendar or daily planner.
- Set a timer at your workplace to remind yourself to take a short walk several times a day.
- Stock a pair of walking shoes in various locations. Keep them in your car, at your workplace, and by the door at home.
- Post your weekly activity log on your refrigerator.
- Use your step counter. Give yourself step challenges: so many steps by lunch, so many steps by the end of the workday, so many steps during TV commercials. Make it a game. If you do, you will be the constant winner.

Keep a Positive Spin

Missing a few days of physical activity doesn't mean you flunk the test. Just don't let an "oh, what's the use" negative attitude take over. Negativity can definitely make it more difficult to get back on track.

When you find yourself missing too many days of exercise and lapsing into negative thinking, try to put a positive spin on the situation. We've provided some examples in the chart below.

Negative spin	**Positive spin**
I've missed three straight days of physical activity. I might as well skip activity altogether this week and start fresh next week.	I'll get back into it this afternoon. Four days a week of doing something is better than seven days of not doing anything.
I blew it this week. I'll never be able to make a go of this. I'll just make a New Year's resolution and try again later.	So I've missed a few sessions. Big deal. That's life. It doesn't mean I've failed. I fail only when I stop trying altogether. Now I just need to focus on getting back on track—like today. I only have time for a ten-minute walk, but that will get me back in the groove. The longer I wait, the harder it will be to get back again.

(continued)

Negative spin	Positive spin
It was a tough day at work (or with the kids). Lots of stress and running around. I'm beat. I deserve a break from my physical activity routine.	Physical activity is a great stress reducer. I'll feel better if I take a walk after work (or after the kids go down). It's something my mind and body will be grateful for.
I can't take time away from my family to be active. That's being selfish.	I've got to take care of myself first if I expect to take care of my family. I can include my family in my activity. We can make a daily walk part of our regular routine, and it will be good for all of us. We'll just watch a little less TV.
It's going to be a crazy workweek. I don't have a lot of time for physical activity.	I won't get stuck in that "all or nothing" rut. Even though I don't have time to do all my physical activity at one time, I can get away for five minutes here and there and do some brisk walking in the building. I'm doing it for my own well-being.

They Did It and You Can, Too

Tina's Story

Remember Tina, the hospital nutrition director we introduced in chapter 1? She had lapsed into inactivity over many years and then found her way back to better health just by inserting a bit of walking into her workday. Tina attributed a good deal of the success of her restoration process to the use of the step counter.

The step counter was a centerpiece of Active Living Every Day, a practical and personalized course offered at her hospital (as well as many medical centers around the country) based in part on research conducted at our center.

"The step counter was a great motivator for me. I would put it on first thing in the morning when I got dressed, and then take it off at night just before showering," she said. "As the famous commercial says, 'Don't leave home without it.' Well, I don't leave my house without my step counter. I'll even attach it to my panties when I'm wearing a dress.

"At work I average fifty-five hundred to six thousand steps a day—from the time I arrive until the time I leave. That's about three miles for me. I take the stairs, walk the hallways, walk to the cafeteria, walk around the building during lunch, go downstairs for the mail, and check with my staff. Every step counts.

"By eight in the evening, if I have nine thousand steps, I'll go out and get another thousand. That's my goal, to get ten thousand each and every day."

Tina became so enthusiastic about the Active Living program that she started teaching it at the hospital. "It's wonderful, so easy, and so totally transforming for sedentary people," she said. "I tell the whole world about it."

When she encounters students from her classes in the street, she'll stop them to make sure they have their step counter on. "Even if they come from church they better have it on or they'll hear from me," she said. "If you make an excuse for one day, you'll make one for the next day as well."

Isabel's Story

For fifteen years or so, Isabel had become increasingly sedentary. A former airline reservation agent and currently a school administrator, she was frequently exhausted at the end of her workday. She once complained to a doctor that she was totally exhausted just from walking up two short flights of stairs to the break room at school. The doctor thought she might have a low iron problem.

Isabel also had had a bout with cancer, and for eight years suffered from "horrible" migraines at least once or twice a month, and sometimes even more. Her doctor said the migraines were not hormone related and gave Isabel some painkilling medication to deal with the problem.

In 2006 she noticed that a colleague, who often complained about the same kind of daily tiredness, suddenly stopped using the *T* word.

"I asked her what was going on," recalled Isabel. "She was looking perkier, as well. She told me that she was using a step counter and that it had given her more energy and a new lease on life. So I decided to look into it."

Isabel called our center for more information. She purchased a step counter. For three days, she wrote down her total daily steps—an average of 5,200 steps.

"I did that much because I had to do some walking around the school during my daily activities," Isabel told us.

She then set up weekly goals to increase her steps. Instead of going directly from point A to point B on campus during the school day, she would go the roundabout way, and she started walking in a nearby park after work.

Her current daily average: 17,000 to 18,000! We asked Isabel about her results.

"After about a week, I started feeling more energy. After a month or so, I noticed I hadn't had a migraine. And to this day, four months later, I still haven't had a migraine. My clothes fit better. That makes me happy, as it would any other woman. And my kids are really proud of me. One of my teenage boys actually volunteered to do the dinner dishes a few times so that I would be able to get in my walk. Sometimes they join me, one on his bike, the other running ahead.

"After I started feeling better, I became more conscious about my diet. Why should I do only one thing right and not give attention to something as important as food? I cut out a lot of sweets."

Enthusiastic about her newfound well-being, Isabel has become something of a step counter ambassador. She has already converted one of her sedentary friends, and she gave a step counter to an overweight nephew as a graduation gift.

"It was the most meaningful thing I could give him," she said.

Richard's Story

Richard, one of our patients, is a computer programmer, which is a highly sedentary profession. He's in his fifties and has always been physically active and had a good level of fitness. His medical tests have always been on the bright side, but in 2005 his numbers took a big leap to a still healthier level.

"What's going on with you?" we asked. "What are you doing that's different? Are you exercising more?"

"No," he said.

"Did you change your diet?"

"No," he answered. "I was curious about how many steps I was taking during a twenty-four-hour period, so I bought a step counter. I quickly realized that I was physically very inactive outside of my regular exercise routine. So I started to set step goals for myself. When I got home every day, I checked my step counter. If I was short of the goal, I would get up after dinner and walk around the block until I got in my additional thousand or fifteen hundred steps to meet my goal. It could be just a ten-, fifteen-, or twenty-minute walk."

Richard found that the extra walk was usually necessary for him to meet his goal. And as a very goal-oriented individual, he made it a point to meet the challenge.

Richard had an appointment with us for an annual checkup about eight months after starting this routine. He absolutely topped off every health parameter that we checked, just by making one simple change.

Here's a person who was already fit, but by doing a bit more, became even healthier. His payoff was big, but the payoff is even bigger when you go up a notch to moderate fitness from being sedentary and unfit. Using the step counter can get you there easily and in practically no time.

7

Move Yourself Plan A Nutrition

> We are all dietetic sinners; only a small percent of what we eat
> nourishes us; the balance goes to waste and loss of energy.
> —Sir William Osler, M.D.

Sometimes unhealthy patients and study participants surprise us and
make multiple and positive lifestyle changes practically overnight.
For one reason or another they see big health problems coming, get
scared, and do an abrupt turnaround. Cold turkey. They'll start a physical activity program, adopt a healthier diet, and begin to effectively deal
with the stress in their lives.

Most, however, have difficulty taking on too much change at once.
It's too stressful. For us at the Cooper Clinic, we'll jump for joy and toss
confetti when a stubbornly sedentary patient gets moving and sustains a
physical activity program.

What if that same person has a poor diet and needs to make a lot of
better food choices for his or her own good? Do we push hard for a
major dietary makeover? Not if we feel we will jeopardize the momentum—and the benefits—of their new resolve to be physically active. In
our experience, simultaneously introducing another big lifestyle change
such as diet and a tedious food plan can easily create a stressful overload. Instead, we prefer to use the easy-does-it, bit-by-bit approach. Just
as we see health improving step-by-step, so do we see gradual benefits
when someone starts eating better bite by bite. There's an old saying,
"Yard by yard, life is hard. Inch by inch, life's a cinch."

Our approach is first to get you up and moving, and sticking with it. At the moment we would like to focus just on your physical activity—stepping forward, using the step counter—and improving your health and fitness status.

Eating Pattern Assessment

After a month or so into the program, when physical activity has become part of your routine, we invite you to look at your diet to see where you can start making some improvements. The eating pattern assessment chart below will help you do that. It was developed at our center to help patients evaluate their diet—what they are doing right and what needs improvement.

For each of the food groups in the chart below, circle the foods you usually eat from that particular category.

Food Group	One	Two	Three
Bread, cereals, and other starchy foods	Whole grain breads, cereals, crackers, and pasta; wild and brown rice; corn tortillas; beans prepared with healthy or limited fats	White bread; presweetened cereal; granola; white rice; regular pasta; cornbread; muffins; regular crackers; flour tortillas; beans prepared with fat	Doughnuts; biscuits; croissants; pastries; egg noodles; high-fat crackers; refried beans; potato skins; French fries; pasta, potatoes, and rice prepared with butter, cream, or cheese
Fruits and vegetables	4 or more servings* of vegetables per day; 2 or more servings* of fruits per day	2–4 servings* per day of combined vegetables and fruit; canned fruit in heavy syrup	Less than 2 servings* of fruits and vegetables a day; coconut; vegetables cooked with cream, butter, or cheese
Dairy products	Skim or 1% milk; 1% yogurt; low-fat soy milk; nonfat cheese; cheese with less than 3 grams of fat per ounce	Reduced fat (2%) milk; 2% yogurt; reduced-fat cheese; light cream cheese; light sour cream	Whole milk; whole milk yogurt; custard-style yogurt; regular sour cream; cream cheese; regular cheeses like ricotta, Swiss, American, cheddar

(continued)

Food Group	One	Two	Three
Meats, poultry, fish, eggs	Small to moderate portions of lean beef and pork tenderloin; extra lean hamburger; skinless poultry; seafood; fish; egg whites or only a few eggs a week	Larger portions of lean beef and pork cuts; lean hamburger; ground turkey; poultry with skin	Marbled beef and pork; regular hamburger; bacon; sausage; bologna; hot dogs; fried chicken; fried fish; canned fish packed in oil; more than 6 egg yolks a week
Fats and oils	Use vegetable oils in moderation when preparing foods. Consume moderate amounts of nuts, avocado, and olives. No trans fats.	Often add fats and oils when preparing foods at home. Use soft margarine.	Always add fats and oils when preparing foods at home. Do not measure the amount of oil used. Frequently eat fried foods and fast foods. Use butter or stick margarine.
Desserts and snacks	Pretzels; angel food cake; fig bars; graham crackers; low-fat crackers and cookies; low-fat popcorn; non-fat plain frozen yogurt without added sugar or fructose; sorbet	Low-fat chips; cakes; brownies; regular popcorn; sherbet	Regular potato, corn, and cheese chips; ice cream; candy; rich cakes; cookies; pies
Beverages	Water; less than 1 or 2 cups of coffee a day; 100% fruit juice; 100% vegetable juice; a variety of tea; little or no alcohol	A few alcoholic beverages; sports drinks; fruit punch	More than 2 cups of coffee a day; more than 2 drinks a day of: regular latte drinks, regular soft drinks, and hot chocolate
Eating away from home	Eat out fewer than 2 times per week	Eat out 2 to 4 times per week	Eat out more than 4 times per week

*One serving = 1 medium piece of fruit; ½ cup chopped or cooked fruits or vegetables; ¾ cup fruit or vegetable juice; 1 cup raw leafy greens.

Interpreting the Results

Into which column (One, Two, or Three) do most of your circled foods fall? If your answers are in . . .

Column one: Congratulations. You are enjoying a healthful diet that may help reduce many of your risk factors for heart disease and stroke. Keep up the good work.

Columns one and two: You are doing a good job of eating a healthful diet. Make a few more changes so that more of your food choices are from column one.

Column two: Your diet is moderately healthy. You may have made some steps in the right direction. Keep making changes slowly until most of your food choices are from column one.

Columns two and three: Your diet is not as heart healthy as it could be. Try to move away from some foods in column three and eat them only once in a while. Make changes slowly so that more of your choices are from column two, then mostly from column one.

Column three: Your diet has room for improvement. Choose one or two food groups and start to slowly make changes toward column two, then column one. Save the column three foods for eating on special occasions.

What works for many people is to slowly start incorporating some healthier foods into their diet. Add an extra piece of fruit here and an extra vegetable there. Eat fewer of the downright unhealthy foods. Making a few changes can gradually take you to a higher level of health—just by doing some simple, commonsense things and not trying to adhere to a rigid diet plan.

Regardless of what you eat, you will still gain multiple benefits from physical activity.

If you want still more guidance on food choices, see our recommendations in chapter 12. Or, if you think you are up to following a comprehensive eating program, we suggest you obtain a copy of *Healthy Eating Every Day* (Human Kinetics, 2005), written by Cooper Aerobics Center nutritional researchers Ruth Ann Carpenter and Carrie Finley. The book is available through online book vendors or through our store (on the Internet at www.coopercomplete.com/books.php, or by phone at 800-393-2221).

Move Yourself
Plan B

Balance Your Approach

Plan B takes you to a higher state of fitness, and the additional health benefits that come with it, through a balanced program of regular, dedicated, and more intense physical activity. At this level you step up to the concept of exercise. It's the next level to move up to if you have incorporated and sustained a program of physical activity in your lifestyle as we laid out in Plan A, or if you are already a regular exerciser but want to hone your fitness in a more effective and comprehensive way.

If you are currently inactive, do *not* start at this level. You can hurt yourself. Go back to Plan A.

Plan B comprises four parts: aerobics, strengthening, stretching, and nutrition.

8

Stepping It Up

People who are successful at exercising regularly don't stop to think about it—they really just do it.
—Sandra Cousins, professor of physical education, University of Alberta

Plan B stands for Balance, a principle that many people neglect in their pursuit of fitness. It is not meant to be a specific workout program, although we present some effective routines for you to get started with in this section. Our primary objective at this point is to show you how to structure cardio, strength, and flexibility workouts yourself, using the same principles we teach our patients and exercise study participants.

First, we'd like you to consider your current activity practice.

Does it emphasize just one element—cardio, strength, or flexibility—at the expense of others?

Is your constant emphasis on a specific program aggravating some part of your body (such as your knee) and keeping you in pain?

Are you doing just cardio? That is the case for many people. It's wonderful exercise, but by itself it may not be good enough. You may play tennis and then go to the gym and work out on the elliptical machine. This combination of activity brings diminished returns because it's pretty much all directed to your cardiorespiratory fitness. Instead, you should set aside some time to improve your strength.

Are you doing just strength training? That's a common guy thing, to get strong. The typical man we see in our fitness center likes to lift weights, and has been doing it since high school. He isn't interested in cardio. He doesn't want to run. We tell the guys that it's okay not to run, but they have to do something aerobically, to maintain the vitality of their heart and lungs.

Are you doing just stretching? We have many women who come to our fitness center for a yoga class every morning. One day we asked a group of them if they were doing anything else besides the yoga. Most answered in the negative. We find this typical of many women. They also would benefit from some cardiovascular fitness and strength training, such as lifting light weights for 15 minutes after their class a few times a week, as well as doing elliptical or stationary bike cardio twice a week for 15 minutes.

It is not necessary for you to join a gym, but wherever and however you decide to increase your fitness level, we would like you to keep variety in mind. A balanced approach yields better overall health benefits.

What's the Best Exercise Program?

That's a question we are asked frequently. The answer: whatever works best for you.

When stepping up your activity level, consider your personal situation. Where do you live and what do you want to do? Do you live in the country where there is no health club nearby? Do you live in the city? Do you want to join a health club? Do you have any equipment? Do you want to purchase any equipment? Do you have a stationary bike or a treadmill at home? Would you consider buying a set of inexpensive dumbbells (they don't have to be heavy) and doing some simple lifting in the house?

All these are personal choices. The most important thing is that you pursue regular physical activity, and if you want to do more, be sure to do it right. It doesn't have to be complicated, just done in a way that is safe and effective for you.

Aerobics and Beyond

The term *aerobic* goes back to the famous French biologist Louis Pasteur to describe microorganisms that live in the presence of oxygen. The word is a combination of the Greek words *aero* (for air) and *bios* (for life). The term *aerobics* (with an *s* at the end) goes back to Kenneth Cooper's 1968 best seller *Aerobics*, which popularized the practice of jogging for health. Applied to exercise, the word means physical activities that improve cardiorespiratory fitness; namely, repetitive and sustained activities such as fast walking, running, swimming, cycling, and cross-country skiing that engage the large muscle groups and enhance the ability of the lungs, heart, and blood vessels to transport oxygen throughout the body.

Aerobic fitness is profoundly protective against premature death from cardiovascular disease and several major cancers. The lion's share of the scientific evidence for that has been developed here at our center, by our own researchers or by researchers around the world using our database. And the vast majority of studies conducted on exercise and health have been done with aerobic activity, even though strength training is of great importance. Aerobic exercise, in particular, pushes blood flow, causes arterial dilation, drops blood pressure, improves good cholesterol, decreases blood fats, enhances the body's usage of blood sugar, encourages better sleep, and benefits all the quality-of-life issues we have discussed in the book. Aerobic exercise impacts every cell of your body.

At our Cooper Aerobics Center campus in North Dallas we have a one-mile-long rubberized track weaving through the thirty-acre grounds. Most any time of the day you will encounter patients, gym members, or staffers churning up mile upon mile on that track. As enthusiastic runners, we ourselves have logged plenty of miles on the track as well. But that's not all we, our patients, or our gym members routinely do.

In the early 1990s, Dr. Cooper and his staff of exercise and medical experts began to realize that aerobics, while fantastic for your heart and cardiovascular fitness, is not enough for overall health and fitness. It is a big part of the exercise package, but not the whole thing.

Our experts began reporting a disturbing development among some of the most aerobically fit patients, especially the older ones. These were people dedicated to the practice of aerobic exercise for cardiovascular health. While they could pass their treadmill tests with flying colors during checkups, the aging process was not treating them as favorably as expected.

Many of these aging patients had become somewhat weak and predisposed to injury. They were losing muscle mass despite their aerobic conditioning.

Why, having spent years following our advice on aerobic exercise, would they now have difficulty with yard work or recreational activities such as snow skiing?

Why had previously uninjured muscles and tendons become problematic?

Why had even their aerobic fitness performance, while excellent compared to most people their age, declined in spite of ongoing, consistent exercise? They found that they could not run as fast, swim as hard, or cycle as sprily as before.

Surely some changes could be explained away by aging, but what was happening to these folks seemed to be more significant. Our experience showed us that successful aging—indeed, successful fitness—requires a number of things, including good nutrition, appropriate stress management, good emotional health, and a well-balanced approach to physical activity. When it comes to total health and fitness, aerobics is just not enough. Strength and flexibility training are needed as well. We can't just *move it*. We need to *move it, lift it, and stretch it!*

This was the conclusion made by our experts. They found that across all age groups of men and women, individuals without a basic level of muscular strength and flexibility are less able to perform the various activities of daily living that are essential for self-sufficiency and living life to the fullest.

With the realization that more than just aerobics is necessary to help our patients engage fully and for as long as possible in life, our center developed a balanced and broadened exercise concept. When we first started suggesting that people didn't need to run long distances—but in fact needed to back off and do other things, namely some strength work and stretching—we received considerable flak from the running world.

Nevertheless, we have fully adopted the balanced and expanded approach. We now send patients to our exercise physiologists to go over strength and stretching techniques. The outcomes from this expanded exercise approach have been astounding at our center. We see patients becoming not only aerobically fit, but stronger and more flexible as well. They undergo head-to-toe improvements in physical conditioning that translate to a greater sense of well-being and ability to carry out daily tasks. They become more fit for life.

Dan's Story

Dan has followed Dr. Cooper's aerobic advice since his twenties. His work as a ship's pilot requires that he remain both physically fit and mentally alert. Regular exercise has been tremendously helpful for that purpose.

When Dan reached fifty about ten years ago, he sought new exercise challenges. He and his wife, also a fitness enthusiast, had made annual treks to a mountain resort in Utah. They prided themselves on hiking with people half their age to the top of the toughest trails. These annual outings continued to keep him feeling young both physically and emotionally, and reinforced his belief in aerobic exercise.

However, Dan began noticing some changes. Chronic knee problems had gradually made running too painful, so he resigned himself to brisk walking, keeping the distances long, and when possible, going higher and higher on hikes to raise the aerobic challenge. He found that the hike to the top of the trails was not as easy as it had been previously in spite of continued, consistent aerobic exercise. While he could still keep up with the best of them, Dan was feeling the difference. Nevertheless, he wanted new challenges. Therefore, in 2002 he planned and completed a trek up Mount Kilimanjaro in east Africa.

During a checkup after the hike, Dan was elated. He said he had been able to complete the trek, while others in his group had turned back. But the climb had worsened the pain in both of his knees and he decided to consult an orthopedic surgeon. The specialist recommended physical therapy and injections into his knees. Dan chose to forgo the injections, but he did go through the physical therapy. The therapist treating him suggested he begin stretching and strengthening the muscles around both knees. We previously had discussed the need for him to do this, but he had resisted. Now he was open to it.

After completing physical therapy, Dan continued to strengthen and stretch the muscles around his knees. The benefits he received, including decreased pain, encouraged him to begin a general strength-training program, using some simple exercises. He continued to exercise aerobically, but his program now contained the added elements of strength and flexibility. He called to say he had made great improvement, and announced that in summer 2003 he was taking on his next big physical challenge: Mount Shasta in northern California!

Dan came in for a checkup six weeks after his Shasta climb and admitted that he never could have completed it without the strength and flexibility training.

"I have always been fit, but I had no idea how much muscle strength and flexibility I had lost, particularly in my upper body," he said. "While Kilimanjaro was tough, it was still mostly aerobic for me. Mount Shasta was a different story. It required more technical climbing, using ice picks and ropes. Had I not strengthened my muscles and made them more limber, I would never have reached the summit. A man and woman who were obviously in good shape—and much younger than me—were not able to complete the ascent. They were aerobically fit, but not strong enough. The Shasta trip was hard for me because I was using muscles I had only recently strengthened, which made it obvious to me how important this part of my fitness program is."

Clearly, climbing different mountains demands different types of physical fitness. The same can be said about our day-to-day lives. Hustling through an airport to make a flight, pushing and pulling a lawnmower around the yard, lifting groceries out of a deep car trunk all require fitness, but each activity requires a different type of fitness. One is not more important than the other; they are all part of the same package.

You don't have to be like Dan and climb far-flung mountaintops. However, if you wish to live a fully active, fully engaged, and fully fruitful life for as long as possible, a balanced exercise regimen is your best ticket.

What—Me Lift Weights?

We hear that comment from many people, particularly women. If you haven't done it before, you may well hesitate at the thought of strength training. The program we prescribe, however, is not designed to create bulging biceps. Far from it. You don't have to pump tons of iron, or even any iron at all. You can make yourself stronger with or without weights, and in the process build up lean muscle mass vital for balance, glucose metabolism, weight control, and bone health. In a very simple way you can improve your core body strength and your major muscle groups and enhance your ability to carry out everyday routines. On top of that, strength training tones your muscles and makes you look good.

In chapter 10, we lay out a basic routine to be done at your own individual level of ability—in the gym or at home—that can help prevent the kind of muscle deterioration we observed with our aging runners.

Stretch It Out

In chapter 11, we present an equally simple but effective stretching program designed to improve your flexibility and prevent injuries. Older tendons and muscles are less pliable and therefore less forgiving when they are challenged by the rigors of exercise. To help them along, you need to pay attention to those activities that enhance their ability to absorb the forces you apply during aerobic and strength exercises. These activities require basic flexibility, and aging does its best to rob us of this. Older athletes will tell you that when they don't stretch as they need to, they tend to ache more. Stretching works the big muscles—the hamstrings, quads, lower back, belly, and shoulder girdle—and makes them more flexible. People of any age who stretch find that they suffer fewer injuries as well as less soreness from exercise and from daily activities such as gardening or even cleaning the house.

Nirvana or Bust?

In the next chapter, we will cover the most popular cardio activities: walking, jogging, swimming, and cycling.

Although we champion a balanced approach to exercise, we acknowledge that not everybody will want to do all three kinds of exercise, or to do them all consistently. To these individuals we say: if you can only do one thing, do the cardio. Is that a complete program? No. Nirvana is about perfection, and we certainly would like to have you following a Nirvana-like aerobic, strength, and stretching routine. But if you can't, you can't. Don't chastise yourself for it. And certainly don't stop the good activity you do, even if it's not a perfect program. There are enough sedentary people out there who throw out the good, or don't even consider it, because they found something better in the form of their Oreos and the TV remote. If you can only do one thing for your health, do the aerobics.

FIT (Frequency, Intensity, and Time)

The programs we have set up in the following chapters are designed to get you started in the right direction with a balanced exercise routine. After you have followed our structured programs for a while, we hope you won't need them anymore. Instead, we hope you will follow the principle of FIT: frequency of sessions, intensity of sessions, and time per session.

You can apply FIT anywhere you are, whether at home or on a business trip or on vacation. It works whether you are a doctor, carpenter, secretary, schoolteacher, or working mother. After you read our ideas and launch yourself into activity—at whatever level works best for you—you will soon be able to take the basic principles and adapt them to your unique situation.

FIT is a simple but profound concept for developing fitness. The FIT approach preconditions muscles, tendons, and ligaments—the structural tissues in the body that support movement—for developing a higher state of fitness. It's like building a house. First you need a strong foundation.

Frequency

The first thing to focus on is how often you exercise. The idea is to establish the habit of regular exercise, keeping your intensity low in the beginning. Later you can build up your momentum comfortably, and keep building it up week after week, month after month, year after year.

Most people tend to work out infrequently and hard (with high intensity). That's precisely the wrong approach. You don't want to become overwhelmed, especially if you are transitioning from Plan A to Plan B. And you certainly don't want to injure yourself by pushing unconditioned muscles and tendons beyond their capabilities.

For the beginner, the routine can be as easy as just walking in the morning or evening and doing some simple stretches while sitting and watching TV. Start with a simple program—perhaps 20 minutes of walking or other cardio three times a week, along with some stretching.

Gradually, as you feel comfortable with the level of activity, add 20 minutes of strength training on alternate days. If you can't do 20 minutes right away, start with 5, 10, or 15 minutes. If you can't work out five days a week, then do it Monday, Wednesday, and Friday.

Ultimately you want to try to get in aerobic activity every day. But in the beginning, your goal is to establish the exercise habit at a level that works for you.

Time

Next you want to increase the length of time you exercise, while maintaining the frequency. If you have gotten comfortable with 15 minutes of walking, five days a week, increase it to 20 minutes, five days a week. At this point, you still don't want to rev up the intensity. Once you feel established with 20 minutes per session, consider moving up to 30 minutes per session.

Keep in mind your ultimate goal of at least 150 minutes of aerobic activity during the course of a week. If you are unable to amass enough aerobic minutes during the week, try to make up for it on weekends with a long walk, hike, or bike ride. For many people, Saturday mornings offer a good opportunity to accumulate a lot of activity.

Intensity

Once you get the frequency and time where they need to be, then, and only then, increase the intensity. Let's say that after a while you are walking 30 minutes a day and covering a mile and a quarter in that time frame. The following week, step up to a mile and a half in the same time frame. You are now increasing intensity, picking up the pace.

. . .

Beginners can start strength training a few weeks after they begin the aerobics program. We outline a simple strength startup program in chapter 10. If you want to go beyond that, it's advisable to seek the guidance of an experienced fitness trainer.

Stretching doesn't require much preconditioning. If you start doing some gentle stretching right away, you will find that your flexibility will improve rapidly. We have provided some easy stretches in chapter 11.

If you have a higher degree of fitness to start with, you can combine all three types of exercise together right at the start.

Below are some sample schedules of how you might want to carry out a month's worth of exercise.

FREQUENCY

	Week 1	Week 2	Week 3	Week 4
Aerobics	Monday, Wednesday, and Friday			
Strength	Tuesday, Thursday			
Stretching	Most days			

INTENSITY

	Week 1	Week 2	Week 3	Week 4
Aerobics	Easy (light sweat, heart and breathing rates increased slightly)		Moderate (breathing slightly heavy but able to converse in short sentences)	
Strength	12–15 repetitions per set			
Stretching	30 seconds per stretch			

TIME

	Week 1	Week 2	Week 3	Week 4
Aerobics	5 minutes	10 minutes	20 minutes	At least 30 minutes
Strength	1 set each exercise		2 sets each exercise	
Stretching	30 seconds per stretch			

Protect Your Aging Joints

Could a more intense exercise and fitness routine, heaven forbid, contribute to arthritis, the painful, potentially crippling disease that wears away the joints?

The answer is maybe. On the one hand, there is no evidence that exercise per se causes arthritis. In fact, we believe strongly that regular non-traumatic exercise acts protectively against the development of arthritis. It helps to build stronger joints and to keep one's weight down. On the other hand, rigorous physical activity involves overuse and extra stress for many joints in the body. There's some risk in that.

For the sake of your joints, and for your body in general, once you get past the age of thirty-five, it's no longer a wise idea to exercise the way you did when you were twenty. As you enter and move through your middle years, you need to exercise smarter and think in *body-friendly* terms. That means listening to your body more, and changing your attitude about exercise.

If you haven't done it already, it's time to scrap the old "no pain, no gain" philosophy. For you men reading this, playing through pain was the macho thing in high school or college, but now it could be a liability, a prescription for injury and joint problems down the road.

The body is made to move in certain directions and planes. This is one reason that, when you develop a physical activity program, particularly with strength training involved, it needs to be balanced.

Joints can incur two types of trauma:

1. *Acute macrotrauma.*   This might occur when you are playing on the basketball court and somebody bangs you from behind and you tear a knee ligament or rip a meniscus. Or if you take a fall and break a bone when you are skiing. In many activities there are plenty of opportunities to strain your muscles, tendons, and joints, and break your bones.

We find acute macrotrauma occurring frequently among weekend warriors, individuals who don't do any regular conditioning or exercise that will make them healthy or more fit. They might meet with their buddies every other weekend to play pickup basketball. That's not the same as being physically active, although many think it is. Guys who do that often sustain macrotrauma injuries.

2. *Repetitive microtrauma.*   Microscopic damage can occur to soft tissue supporting joints from repetitive exercise; that is, doing the same activity over and over. The result over time is bursitis and tendonitis.

One of the problems we see is caused by unbalanced strength training. We call it the "shaving mirror workout" where (this is mostly a guy thing again) you only work the "ego" muscles you see in the mirror. That means doing lots of push-type exercises such as bench presses, curls, and push-ups.

The rule of thumb for weight training is that for every *push* exercise you do, you need to do a *pull* exercise. If you do a bicep curl, you need to do a triceps extension. You should work opposite muscle groups as well so you don't create irregular forces—too strong on one side, too weak on the other—that move the joints. A common cause of rotator cuff shoulder problems is doing just push-ups. You develop anterior deltoid muscles that are Cadillacs, and muscles in the back that are Volkswagens. So you tug everything forward and misalign the joints. Inappropriate exercising of muscles can aggravate joints.

If you had an injury to a joint earlier in life—say, from playing high school or college sports—you are at higher risk to develop arthritis in that same joint later on in life, and even as early as middle age. If this describes your situation, you should definitely consult a sports medicine doctor or an orthopedist before embarking on an exercise program after a long layoff.

One of the big problems among athletic middle-aged men is that they still follow a weight-training program taught to them by their coaches in high school. The routine may produce a good effect, but it may be totally incorrect biomechanically and potentially risky to the joints.

The Danger of All or Nothing

The following story is a good example of how you can get into trouble by violating the FIT principle.

George is a sixty-seven-year-old dentist who suffered with the nagging chronic lower back pain that afflicts many in his profession. We see many dentists in our clinic with neck and back problems stemming from hours every day stooping over patients, sometimes at very odd angles.

George had always been an athlete, an accomplished cyclist. As with

many men, however, his mind-set was stuck on exercise for performance, not activity for health. A few months prior to the cycling season,
George would hit the road on his bike. He would gradually crank up the
mileage to reach the conditioning he needed for competition. Then,
when the racing season was over, he would put the bicycle away until
the next year, stop the intense training, and only do some inconsistent
and inadequate exercise.

In the beginning, his back problem seemed to surface only during the
off season. Over time, however, the discomfort continued throughout
the year, even during training, and became progressively more painful.
By age sixty-four, George decided to have lower back surgery to correct
the problem, which was diagnosed as bulging disks. He was extremely
disappointed that he needed an operation because he thought that his
cycling activity would have protected him.

The surgery did alleviate his pain. However, had George kept active
in the off season—maintaining a healthy body as well as a semblance of
conditioning—he may have been able to delay or minimize the disk
problem. The annual stress of intense training and racing would likely
not have been so hard on his aging and otherwise inactive body. Com-
petitive cycling, like other sports, requires that the muscles of the body
be conditioned as well as the cardiorespiratory system. We advised
George to train consistently in the off season, not as hard as during the
cycling season, utilizing a program of moderate stationary cycling along
with some simple back exercises.

The combination of surgery and correct conditioning worked for
George. He was able to continue practicing both in the profession and
the competition he enjoys. He made an impressive and pain-free return
to his master's cycling competitions stronger than ever.

By improving his conditioning program, George enhanced the functional state of the muscles required to maximally perform the movements of cycling. By conditioning year-round, and addressing the
body's biomechanics, he was able to improve even at an older age. That
is the primary point behind working out smarter, not harder!

Work with a Qualified Trainer

An integrated physical activity program can be started at any age. If you
have been sedentary for a long period of time, once you attain a mini-

mum level of fitness such as we recommend in Plan A, there is no reason you can't step up. But please check with your physician first if you want to make that upward move.

Then consult with a fitness trainer to find the best combined program that works for you. Ideally, talk to a trainer certified by the American College of Sports Medicine (www.acsm.org on the Internet, or call 317-637-9200), the American Alliance for Health, Physical Education, Recreation and Dance (www.aahperd.org on the Internet, or call 703-476-3400), or our own Cooper Institute for Aerobics Research (www.cooperaerobics.com on the Internet, or call 972-233-4832).

Work, at least initially, with an experienced and certified personal trainer. If such a person isn't available, see a physical therapist or a sports medicine specialist, somebody trained in biomechanics. Too often we encounter patients so ingrained in old routines that they resist change. The tendency is to fall back to the same old routine, and that's courting trouble.

Aches and Pains

We often see patients who complain of pain in the knee or back or elsewhere. The reason is that they are violating basic principles of exercise.

Here's an example: A patient comes in complaining about knee pain. He doesn't understand what caused it. It's likely that the person has increased the volume and intensity of his training simultaneously. He might be a cycling enthusiast, for example, who added an extra outing on his bike during the week, but because of time constraints, had to do it more intensely. By modifying his program, he should be able to cool off what has become patellar tendonitis.

If you develop some ongoing aches and pains in a knee, hip, ankle, shoulder, or other joint, how do you know if you have early arthritis or a muscle, ligament, or tendon problem?

We tell our patients in these situations to stop the impact and stress on that particular part of the body for a week to ten days. If we're talking knees, stop jogging, and stop doing any start-stop court sports such as tennis, racquetball, or basketball, which cause a lot of soft-tissue injury. Do some swimming, cycling, or something else to get your weight off the discomfort zone. And take a bit of an anti-inflammatory such as ibuprofen.

At the end of that period if the painful area has improved, that indicates a soft-tissue injury. It's good news. But you may have to restructure your program, because if you go out and do the same old exercise again, you are going to have more problems.

If the area feels better when you're off of it but the discomfort isn't altogether gone, or it's still there with activity, then you probably have something more than just a simple soft-tissue injury. That's the time to get a medical opinion.

The point of all these warnings is not to discourage intense exercise. If you want to go to that level, just do it wisely. The saying "An ounce of prevention is worth a pound of cure" really applies here.

One of our patients is Casey Meyers, now in his late seventies. Always a great exercise enthusiast, Casey was an avid runner for many years. Over time he developed knee arthritis, probably a result of running on concrete in the days before we had more protective shoes.

The arthritis got so bad that Casey needed a knee replacement, first in one knee and then in the other. But that wasn't going to stop him. After his recovery, he became a power walker, and with hard walking alone he maintains superior fitness.

If you are looking for a great book on walking for fitness, check out Casey's book, *Walking: A Complete Guide to the Complete Exercise.*

9

Move It! Do Cardio
for Heart Health

And I love to ride my bike, which is great aerobics, but also just a
great time for me to think, so it's like this terrific double bill.
—Actor Robin Williams

To maximize your Plan B cardio experience, we have laid out fifteen
examples of the most popular aerobic programs: walking, jogging,
swimming, and cycling (including with a stationary bike). They are
divided into beginning, intermediate, and advanced categories. All
incorporate the FIT principles we discussed in the previous chapter.

If you are already a walker, or you walked regularly until six or so
months ago, you might be able to start with the intermediate walking
program. To be sure, however, you may want to test your level of fitness
to determine a comfortable starting level. On your first day, try the
beginning program for Week 1: cover 1.5 miles in 21 minutes. To determine distance accurately, you may want to purchase a pedometer, which
is a step counter that also logs distance. Then go to your nearest high
school running track. Usually they are quarter-mile ovals. Alternatively,
use an indoor running track if you have access to one. Walk the course
to determine how many steps it takes you to complete one mile. Strides
vary from person to person. That way you can personalize your pedometer to your particular stride and program, and gauge your distance no
matter where you walk. Then ask yourself how easy it was. If it was too
easy, the next day take the starting point of the intermediate program:

cover 2 miles in 27:30 minutes. How easy was that? Again, if it was too easy, go to the advanced starting point of 2.5 miles in 33:15 minutes. You can test yourself similarly with any of these activities.

All these programs result in the same improved level of fitness. The main difference between a beginner, intermediate, and advanced program is how fast you move through from start to finish.

Take the walking program as an example. The beginners' program starts at an easier level, but at the end of ten weeks you are covering the same distance (4 miles) in the same time (55 minutes) as the advanced exerciser. The advanced walker starts more intensely. It takes the ten weeks in the beginners' program, seven weeks in the intermediate, and four weeks in the advanced program to achieve the same frequency, intensity, and time. And at this level you have reached the point where you will start losing weight.

If you have a bigger weight- and waist-loss goal in mind, you will want to proceed to Plan C, but don't do it until you have gone through the entire Plan B program. This applies to all cardio activities. The last week of the Plan B program is the jump-off point for Plan C. If you reach this level, you will have attained the conditioning that prepares you, if you choose, for the more intense energy expenditure necessary for effective weight loss.

Plan B Walking Programs

BEGINNER (INCLUDING TREADMILL)

Week	Distance (miles)	Time (minutes)	Frequency/Week (times)
1	1.5	21:00	5
2	2.0	28:45	5
3	2.0	28:30	5
4	2.0	28:00	5
5	2.0	28:00	3
	and 2.5	35:30	2
6	2.5	35:00	3
	and 3.0	43:15	2
7	2.5	34:45	3
	and 3.0	43:00	2
8	2.5	34:30	3
	and 3.0	42:30	2
9	3.0	42:30	5
10	4.0	55:00	5

INTERMEDIATE (INCLUDING TREADMILL)

Week	Distance (miles)	Time (minutes)	Frequency/Week (times)
1	2.0	27:30	5
2	2.0	27:30	3
	and 2.5	33:45	2
3	2.0	27:30	3
	and 2.5	33:30	2
4	2.5	33:15	3
	and 3.0	41:15	2
5	2.5	33:00	3
	and 3.0	40:00	2
6	3.0	41:00	5
7	4.0	55:00	5

ADVANCED (INCLUDING TREADMILL)

Week	Distance (miles)	Time (minutes)	Frequency/Week (times)
1	2.5	33:15	4
	and 3.0	41:30	1
2	2.5	33:00	3
	and 3.0	40:00	2
3	3.0	41:00	5
4	4.0	55:00	5

Plan B Jogging Programs

BEGINNER (WALK/JOG)

Week	Activity	Distance (miles)	Time (minutes)	Frequency/Week (times)
1	Walk	1.0	18:00	5
2	Walk	1.5	24:00	5
3	Walk/Jog	1.5	20:30	5
4	Walk/Jog	1.5	19:30	5
5	Walk/Jog	1.5	18:30	3
6	Jog	1.0	10:45	2
	Jog	1.5	17:30	3
7	Jog	1.0	10:15	2
	Jog	1.5	16:30	3
8	Jog	1.0	9:45	3
	Jog	1.5	15:30	2
9	Jog	1.0	9:15	3
	Jog	1.5	14:55	2
10	Jog	1.0	8:55	3
	Jog	2.0	20:30	2
11	Jog	1.0	8:45	2
	Jog	1.5	13:00	2
	Jog	2.0	20:00	1
12	Jog	2.0	20:00	5

INTERMEDIATE (WALK/JOG)

Week	Activity	Distance (miles)	Time (minutes)	Frequency/ Week (times)
1	Walk	1.0	18:00	5
2	Walk	1.0	16:00	5
3	Walk/Jog	1.0	14:00	5
4	Walk/Jog	1.0	12:00	5
5	Walk/Jog	1.5	18:00	5
6	Walk/Jog	1.5	17:00	5
7	Jog	1.5	16:00	5
8	Jog	1.5	15:00	5
9	Jog	2.0	22:00	5
10	Jog	2.0	20:00	5

ADVANCED (WALK/JOG)

Week	Activity	Distance (miles)	Time (minutes)	Frequency/ Week (times)
1	Walk	1.0	18:00	5
2	Walk/Jog	2.0	24:00	5
3	Jog	2.0	20:00	5
4	Jog	2.0	20:00	5

Plan B Swimming Programs

BEGINNER

Week	Distance (yards)	Time (minutes)	Frequency/Week (times)
1	300	6:00	5
2	400	8:30	5
3	400	8:30	5
4	400	8:00	2
	and 500	10:30	3
5	400	8:00	2
	and 600	12:30	3
6	500	10:30	3
	and 700	14:30	2
7	600	12:00	4
	and 800	16:30	1
8	600	11:30	3
	and 800	16:00	2
9	800	15:30	4
10	1,000	19:30	5

INTERMEDIATE

Week	Distance (yards)	Time (minutes)	Frequency/Week (times)
1	400	8:30	5
2	400	8:00	2
	and 500	10:30	3
3	400	8:00	2
	and 600	12:30	3
4	600	12:30	4
	and 800	16:30	1
5	600	12:30	3
	and 800	16:00	2
6	800	15:30	4
7	1,000	19:30	5

ADVANCED

Week	Distance (yards)	Time (minutes)	Frequency/Week (times)
1	500	10:30	3
	and 700	14:30	2
2	600	12:30	3
	and 800	16:30	2
3	800	15:30	4
4	1,000	19:30	5

Plan B Cycling Programs

Most stationary bikes use MPH as the determinant of intensity (in other words, faster speeds = higher intensity). A few brands, like the Schwinn Airdyne, use a "load" factor to gauge intensity. For those models, follow the intensity guidelines we have described in the previous chapter (in the FIT discussion). Work out at a load sufficient to cause perspiration and increased breathing, but not so intense that you couldn't carry on a conversation in short sentences.

BEGINNER (STATIONARY OR OUTDOOR)

Week	Speed (MPH)	Time (minutes)	Frequency/Week (times)
1	10	5:00	5
2	10	7:30	5
3	12	10:00	5
4	12	12:30	5
5	12	14:00	5
6	15	14:00	5
7	18	14:00	5
8	18	16:00	5
9	18	20:00	5
10	18	24:00	5
11	18	27:00	5
12	20	30:00	5

INTERMEDIATE (STATIONARY OR OUTDOOR)

Week	Speed (MPH)	Time (minutes)	Frequency/Week (times)
1	10	7:30	5
2	10	10:00	5
3	12	14:00	5
4	15	14:00	5
5	18	14:00	5
6	18	20:00	5
7	18	24:00	5
8	18	27:00	5
9	18	30:00	5
10	20	30:00	5

ADVANCED (STATIONARY OR OUTDOOR)

Week	Speed (MPH)	Time (minutes)	Frequency/Week (times)
1	12	12:00	5
2	15	14:00	5
3	18	20:00	5
4	18	24:00	5
5	18	30:00	5
6	20	30:00	5

10

Lift It! Get Stronger, Not Bulky

Our real problem, then, is not our strength today; it is rather the vital necessity of action today to ensure our strength tomorrow.
—Dwight D. Eisenhower

Most people think strength training means musclemen and women and gut-busting exercises, but that is far from what we have in mind for you. As we explained in chapter 8, Plan B is for health, fitness, and balance. We're not out to turn you into Superman or Superwoman. We just want to give you some guidance for strengthening your muscles simply, safely, and efficiently in order to improve your functional fitness and overall health. Our Plan B program is basic, primarily for a newcomer to the concept of strength training. However, it can be followed long term to improve the strength of the major muscle groups in your body, or it can be used as a conditioning program for more intense weight training later on.

As you will see, most of these routines can be done without any props. You can do them easily at home. A few will be more effective if you use dumbbells, starting with 5 or 10 pounds, or even fewer. Use a weight that you can comfortably lift at the beginning. You can purchase dumbbells at any sporting goods store.

Don't strain yourself to do any of these exercises. Just do what is comfortable for you. Increase the number of repetitions slowly. You're in no hurry and you're not competing with anybody. If you have any medical or physical condition, show these exercises to your doctor before trying them.

In general, when you begin a strength-training program you will experience some slight muscle aches over the next couple of days. The muscle aches should be generalized, and should improve from day to day. Any concentrated pain, or pain in a joint associated with a sensation of instability (like the joint will give way), should be brought to the attention of your trainer or physician.

Upper-Body Muscles

PUSH-UP

It's hard to beat the common push-up for building up the strength of your chest, upper arms, forearms, and trunk muscles. Start by lying flat on the floor, as shown in the picture at the top right.

Now push your upper body up by straightening your arms. Do it slowly, and hold for 5 seconds. Then slowly lower yourself back down. Start with as many repetitions as you can do comfortably, even if it is only one. Then build up slowly. Aim for ten, twenty, or even thirty repetitions over time, or to a level where you feel you have reached a plateau and it's uncomfortable to proceed further.

If you have never done a push-up before, you may want to start with a "beginner" push-up, as illustrated in the picture at the bottom right, with your knees on the floor. Once you can do ten repetitions comfortably, advance to the standard military push-up.

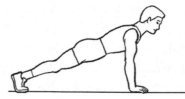

Preparing to do a push-up

"Military" push-up

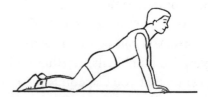

"Beginner" push-up

SHOULDER ABDUCTION—THE BUTTERFLY

This simple exercise builds up the muscles in the front and back of your chest as well as your shoulders. It's an excellent routine for improving posture. If you don't have a bench to lie on, you can put some chairs in a row or even use a table. Start without the dumbbells. After six weeks, progress to using light dumbbells.

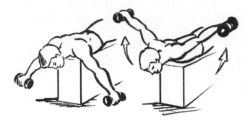

Shoulder abduction

Lie on a bench, belly down. Raise your arms upward. Hold for 5 seconds and then slowly lower. Do ten repetitions. Over time, if desired, progress to more repetitions and heavier weights.

OVERHEAD PRESS

The overhead press extends the elbow and flexes the shoulders, building up the arm and upper chest muscles. Start with a 5-pound dumbbell in each hand, or lighter if 5 pounds is too heavy.

Stand with your arms at your sides and elbows bent, as shown. Reach up overhead and straighten both arms. Hold for 5 seconds. Start with ten repetitions, or whatever number is comfortable for you, and work your way up slowly to twenty-five repetitions. After you reach twenty-five, you can progress, if desired, to heavier dumbbells.

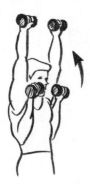

Overhead press

Lower-Body Muscles

QUADRICEPS—EXTENSION AND SQUATS

The quadriceps are a group of muscles located on the front and sides of each thigh. They function to allow the extension of the knee. You want strong quads to protect and maintain normal knee movement. If you have never done any exercises for your quads, we suggest starting with something simple, such as standing up from a sitting position, as shown in the picture below. This exercise strengthens the quads as well as your belly and back-stabilizing muscles.

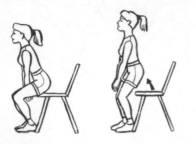

Sitting to standing position (quadriceps extension)

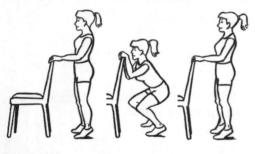

Squats

Start with ten repetitions of sit and stand. Progress to twenty-five. Once you can do twenty-five, advance to the squat exercise, as shown in the picture at the bottom left.

Squats go a ways further and build up not only the thighs and abdominal stabilizers, but also your calf muscles, hamstrings (the muscles in the back of your thigh that help extend the leg at the hip and flex the leg at the knee), and glutes (the muscles in your butt that enable your thigh to move to the rear and sides).

Hold on to a chair and stand on your tiptoes. Squat down to a level where your thigh is at about a 45-degree angle (to what is often referred to as a three-quarter squat). Don't drop down to the same plane as the seat of the chair or the floor. That's too far. Just go to half of that level. Try to stay on your toes as much as possible. Stand back up using the least amount of support from your arms. You want your legs to be doing the work. Start with ten repetitions, if you can, and work up to twenty-five.

HAMSTRING FLEX

Do this exercise after the previous one, also using a chair for support. It may look like hardly anything, but if you do it very slowly and deliberately, you will give your hamstrings an additional simple but efficient workout.

Stand, holding on to the back of a chair. Slowly bend one knee, as shown. Hold for 5 seconds. Slowly lower. Do ten repetitions with each leg, and work up to twenty-five repetitions.

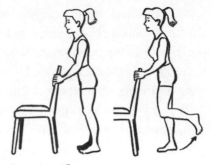

Hamstring flex

STRAIGHT LEG RAISE

This is a two-part exercise. You'll do only the first routine for six weeks, then add the second.

In the first leg raise illustrated at the right you lie on your back with one knee straight and the other bent, as shown. Raise your straight leg to about a 45-degree angle. Hold for 5 seconds and slowly lower it back down. Do ten repetitions. Then repeat

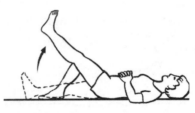

Straight leg raise

with the other leg. This exercise strengthens the front part of the quads, providing support to the knees and the lower abdomen.

After six weeks, add the second leg raise to your routine, illustrated at the bottom right. In this exercise, movements are the same except that now your toes point outward. With your foot in an outward-facing direction, the raising and lowering of the straight leg works the abductor muscle (inner thigh). Again, do ten repetitions with each leg.

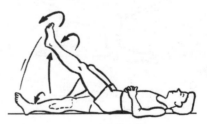

Straight leg raise (with side turn)

Stomach muscles

THE CRUNCH

This classic crunch exercise strengthens and tightens your core midsection muscles. Lie on your back, as shown in the illustration on the next page, with both knees bent. Reach down toward the knees and curl your trunk upward. Hold the position for 5 seconds. Slowly lower your upper body back down. Do ten repetitions and work up to about twenty-five.

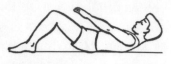

The crunch

When you perform this exercise, don't interlock your fingers behind your head as many people do. You don't want to tug or strain your neck.

Back muscles

BACK EXTENSION

These exercises strengthen your back. As in the illustration below, start in the "Superman" position, face down. Place a 2-inch towel roll under

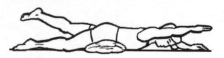

Back extension (beginner)

your forehead and a pillow under your belly. Tighten your buttocks. Raise one arm and the opposite leg (e.g., left arm, right leg). Hold for 5 seconds. Slowly lower. Do ten repetitions. Repeat with the opposite arm and leg.

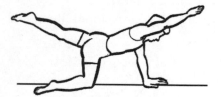

Back extension (advanced)

After six weeks, advance to the next position shown in the picture at the left, using the same right arm-left leg, and then left arm-right leg combinations. Work your way up to twenty-five repetitions.

Get Stronger Safely

We strongly recommend that you make sure you lift correctly and do not hurt your body. If you have any doubts about correct lifting techniques, consult a personal trainer. Even for readers with some experience lifting weights, it's well worth the expense to prevent injury that could possibly plague you for years. You may be someone who once was a high school athlete, has been jogging for the last thirty years, and hasn't lifted weights since school and now wants to start again. Be careful!

Training errors from lifting weights can cause injuries such as muscle and ligament strains and tendonitis. Although improper strength training may or may not contribute to arthritis, middle-aged or older individuals often already have an element of arthritis, and an incorrect technique can aggravate the situation. Thus lifts done when they were young (that they thought were correct) all of a sudden seem to hurt now that they are older. Young, healthy joints allow you to "get away with" training errors. Older joints, ligaments, tendons, and muscles are not nearly as forgiving, and require appropriate training.

Finally, older individuals should avoid heavy lifting (sets where they can only do six to eight repetitions of a particular set), unless they have absolute confidence that their training technique is correct.

Tedd Mitchell's Story

I'm forty-five now, and until about five years ago, I was one of those guys doing those same routines I learned as a high school athlete. Over the years I had maintained a consistent program of exercise and weight training, but when I checked out my technique with a trainer at our center, I got a big surprise.

I was astounded to learn that the way I had been lifting weights for years was probably detrimental. The trainer showed me that my lifting technique on a number of machines was wrong. In the past, my body had been able to tolerate lifting improperly. Now that I was older, it might not be able to. It was time to change.

Like me, you may think you know what you're doing, but you may not. And if you are not, you may be hurting yourself. If you have any doubts about your lifting technique, you are much better off paying for the guidance of an experienced trainer than suffering pain and having to pay the doctor later on.

11

Stretch It! Get Flexible

I never struggled with injury problems because of my preparation—in particular my stretching.
—Two-time Olympic hurdle gold medalist Edwin Moses

Muscles that are growing older are much happier when they get a regular stretching. But there's no need to wait until your later years to make stretching a daily habit. Old or young, male or female, you will feel better and suffer fewer injuries if you keep your muscles flexible. Plan B incorporates a brief stretching routine to follow your regular aerobic and strength workouts.

Many people have the mistaken notion that they should stretch *before* exercising. Bad idea. Stretching cold muscles can lead to tears or injury. Stretch *at the end* of your workout, when your muscles are warmed up and supple, or after about 10 minutes of light aerobic activity, such as walking, bicycling, or stair climbing. Work hard enough to generate a light sweat. When your muscles feel warm, it's safe to stretch.

Here are some other stretching tips:

- A light muscle tension should be felt throughout the stretch. If pain occurs in any joint or muscle, release the stretch.
- Hold each stretch for 20 or 30 seconds. Perform two or three repetitions.

- Don't bounce! Stretch only until you feel resistance, then back off slightly.
- Breathe comfortably.

Below we've provided a stretching routine to get you started.

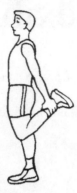

STANDING QUADRICEPS STRETCH

Stand straight, as shown, and grab one ankle. Perform a posterior pelvic tilt, meaning that you tilt backward from the top of the pelvis while squeezing the glute (buttocks) muscles. Feel the tension in the thigh muscle of the leg you are holding. Switch legs.

Standing quadriceps stretch

STRAIGHT LEG STANDING HAMSTRING STRETCH

Stand with one leg elevated and propped up on a table, bench, or chair. Tilt your pelvis forward until you feel a stretch in the hamstrings. Stretch the other leg similarly.

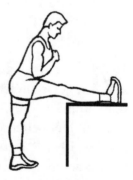

Hamstring stretch

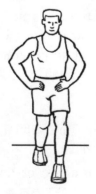

HIP FLEXOR

Assume a staggered stance. Slightly rotate the back leg internally. Draw in your belly button to activate the abdominal stabilizing musculature. Tighten your buttocks and tilt backward from the top of your pelvis (posterior tilt). Don't move your back leg, pull the foot backward, or arch your lower back. Then switch legs. The motion in this exercise occurs mainly with the backward pelvic tilt.

Hip flexor

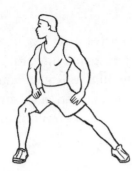

Hip adductor

HIP ADDUCTOR

Position yourself as shown, with one leg straight and the other leg bent, and both feet pointed straight ahead. Draw in your belly button. Slowly tilt your upper body sideways in the direction of the bent leg until you feel tension in the groin area of the straight leg. Switch sides.

CALF-BENT-KNEE STRETCH

Stand close to a wall. Face the wall and lean against it, pressing the palms of the hands against the wall for support. Bring one leg forward for additional support, and raise the heel of the trailing leg as shown. Both feet should point forward. Draw your belly button inward. Lower the heel of your trailing leg so that the foot is now flat, and bend the trailing knee until you feel slight tension in the calf. Keep the rear leg straight. Do not allow the foot or knee to fold inward or roll outward. Switch legs and repeat.

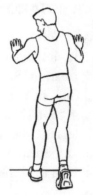

Calf-bent-knee stretch
(starting position)

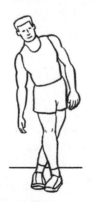

Outer hip abductor stretch
(stretch position)

OUTER HIP ABDUCTOR STRETCH

Stand, as shown, with your left leg crossed behind the right leg. Tilt your upper body sideways and down, until you feel a stretch in the left hip. Switch legs to stretch the right hip.

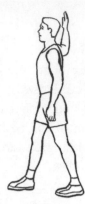

PECTORAL STRETCH

Stand with your side against a wall, forearm flush on the wall with fingers facing upward, as shown. Draw in your belly button. Rotate your trunk slowly forward around the stationary arm until you feel a slight stretch in the front of the shoulder. Switch sides.

Pectoral stretch

NECK ROTATION

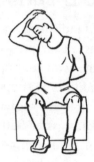

This exercise stretches the important levator scapula muscle, at the back and side of the neck, that permits neck rotation. Sit on a chair. Draw in your belly button. Tuck in your chin and rotate your head toward one of your shoulder tips. At the same time, retract and depress the shoulder on that side. After doing three repetitions on one side, perform the same stretch on the other side.

Neck rotation

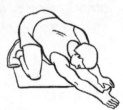

BACK STRETCH

Kneel, as shown, to perform this shoulder and back (latissimus dorsi) stretch. Reach out with one arm. Turn the palm upward (externally rotating the shoulder) and push upward as well with the lower back. Do three repetitions on each side.

Back stretch

MCKENZIE PRESS-UP

This maneuver contributes to normal motion of the spine. Lie on your stomach and place your hands, palms pressing against the

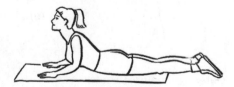

McKenzie press-up (stretch position)

floor, just above the tops of your shoulders. Inhale deeply and start pressing upward (pushing up) slowly. Exhale as you push up. Do not lift your pelvis off the floor. Relax the buttocks and spine muscles. Hold the position at the top, as shown, until you have to take a breath. Inhale as you slowly lower your body back to the starting position. Repeat this exercise ten times. Warning: Do not perform this exercise if you have any lower back discomfort or pain.

SIDE-CROSSED LEG ROTATIONAL

Lie on your back. Pull both your legs up toward your chest, then cross the left leg, as shown, over the right leg. Rotate the lower body to the right. Maintain both shoulder blades in contact with the floor. Perform the same stretch on both sides.

Side-crossed leg rotational

12

Move Yourself Plan B Nutrition

Bigger snacks mean bigger slacks.

—Anonymous

There's nothing complicated about good nutrition. It really is a matter of common sense. For many years we have been teaching commonsense eating to thousands of patients, enabling them to make good nutrition a part of an overall healthy lifestyle. When they leave our center they know how to eat for health, whether they eat at home or frequent restaurants.

On the following pages you will find a distillation of the nutritional education course we teach our patients. We're grateful to Kathy Duran-Thal, R.D., our director of nutrition, for sharing this information. The recommendations are meant to provide a good nutritional accompaniment to a physically active lifestyle. If your goal is to lose substantial weight, you need to follow a specific calorie-restrictive diet, as we detail in Plan C. But first you need to sustain a regular physical activity routine and step up your fitness intensity, as we have outlined here in Plan B. Only then should you attempt Plan C.

At the end of this chapter you will also find some guidelines on using supplements, based on information provided by Conrad Earnest, Ph.D., our former director of human performance and nutrition.

Four Nutritional Golden Rules

Throughout the book we have discussed the many benefits of physical activity. Whatever level of physical activity you are at—whether you're just getting started with Plan A, or upgrading from partial activity to a more intense Plan B approach—these four nutritional golden rules will speed, reinforce, and amplify the benefits of your physical activity. Even if you can make just a few of the changes we recommend, you will see a big difference. Small changes maintained over a lifetime become a lifestyle.

1. Don't Think Diet, Think Healthy Eating

You may be thinking, "What diet are these guys pushing?" A lot of doctors push diets. We don't. We only want you to eat healthfully as a type of behavior, just as doing physical activity is a type of behavior.

The best diet is no diet at all. Why? Because typically people go on a diet until they reach their goal and then they regress to the eating habits that got them in trouble in the first place.

Also, many diets encourage imbalance by restricting or emphasizing a particular food group. This kind of diet is difficult to maintain and over time could become dangerous to your health. Whether you need to lose, gain, or maintain, make healthy eating your priority. Stay balanced.

Following fads such as no-carbohydrate meal plans can upset a healthy balance of calories. High-protein, low-carbohydrate diets can be dangerous to people prone to kidney disease or metabolic disorders.

Food is your source of energy and essential nutrients that your body needs to function. You need enough of many different foods to keep the body running. Chocolate cake is okay as long as you don't overdo it. Sure, everyone wants a treat or something special as a reward. Just make sure not to make it an everyday occurrence.

The American Institute for Cancer Research reports that 78 percent of Americans believe the kind of food they eat is more important for weight management than the amount of food they eat. They would rather cut out entire categories of food from their diets than scale back their overall consumption.

Moderation and variety are the keys to good nutrition and to staying healthy. In your food choices, emphasize quality, not quantity.

2. Concentrate on Complex Carbohydrates

About 45 to 65 percent of what you eat every day should come from plant-derived foods such as fruits, vegetables, whole grains, breads, and cereals. Complex carbohydrates are nature's gift to good nutrition. They are low in fat and calories, cholesterol free, and rich in vitamins, minerals, and fiber.

3. Limit Fats

About 20 to 35 percent of your daily food intake should come from fats. Saturated fats, found primarily in foods of animal origin and in some oils (palm, coconut), can increase cholesterol. This type of fat should make up 10 percent or less of your total fat intake. Think *lean* when it comes to cuts of beef, veal, and pork; eat more fish (a rich source of heart healthy omega-3 fatty acids) and skinless poultry; and choose low-fat or fat-free dairy products.

Trans fat is one type of fat you should avoid. Trans fats are the man-made, partially hydrogenated fats used in processed food to prolong the shelf life of an estimated 75 percent of the food eaten in the standard U.S. diet. They are in margarine and shortening, packaged baked goods, fried foods, frozen products such as fish sticks and French fries, microwavable popcorn, commercial salad dressings, pancake mixes, and more. The list is practically endless.

Since January 2006 food manufacturers have had to reveal the trans fat content on the labels of their products. So be sure to read labels, and make another purchase choice if you see trans fats as ingredients. You should avoid them like the plague. They are linked to cellular damage that causes inflammation, disease, and age-related changes. They promote harmful oxidation of cholesterol and lower your good cholesterol. They also sabotage the body's ability to use good, essential fatty acids—such as fish oil—that have important anti-inflammatory properties.

Not all fats spell trouble; indeed, certain fats are vital for good health, such as the essential omega-3 fatty acids found in fish. We must get polyunsaturated fats (found in corn, soybean, safflower, sunflower, sesame, and cottonseed oils) from what we eat. The body doesn't manufacture them. Without these polyunsaturated fats, there is a risk of problems with the liver, heart, or circulatory system.

Monounsaturated fats, found in olive and peanut oils, are believed to actually help lower your cholesterol.

4. Go Easy on the Protein

Americans used to equate the good life with sitting down to a marbled steak that practically filled the plate. Today having a lean steak that fits in the palm of your hand (3 ounces) is considered eating well. Two 3-ounce servings of protein are all an average adult needs on a daily basis, according to the American Heart Association.

So cut down on animal protein (it contains saturated fats) by using meat as the flavoring in a rice or pasta dish rather than as the focus of a meal. Think of protein not as the star of a meal, but as a supporting actor.

Five Common Nutritional Traps

Changing the way you eat can be quite a challenge. The road is packed with pitfalls. The following tips will help you navigate around five big ones.

1. Overeating

Clearly, a no-brainer. But you'd be surprised how easy it is to overindulge, especially if you watch TV, listen to the radio, read the newspaper, or are busy socializing during a meal. All are activities that seem to override our awareness of satiety—when we've had enough to eat. There's a particularly strong association between eating meals in front of a TV and overeating. Nutritionists routinely remind people interested in losing weight never to eat in front of the TV.

According to ancient Indian wisdom, we should never eat to the point of fullness, only to the point of satisfaction. The advice is thousands of years old, but very relevant in this age of obesity.

2. Skipping Breakfast

Breakfast means "breaking your fast." Keep in mind that food is fuel. We need to fuel up in the morning by eating breakfast, and our fuel should then be able to take us to the next refueling point—lunch. So eat breakfast.

Omitting breakfast places a strain on the body. As a result you may feel more fatigued and irritable, not be able to work as efficiently, and react to things more slowly. You may have a letdown feeling by 10 A.M. Research has also shown a connection between skipped breakfast and a tendency to have more mishaps. When breakfast is adequate, late-morning work production and reaction time are increased.

Another problem with breakfast may be what we are not eating. Include a high-protein food (egg white, yogurt, cottage cheese, low-fat cheese), starch (whole-grain bread, oatmeal, high-fiber cereal), fat (such as nuts), and a piece of fruit for breakfast. These foods should fuel you for approximately four hours. Plan on refueling in four hours for lunch, and again in four to five hours for dinner.

More than 60 million Americans skip breakfast. The two most frequently used excuses are "I don't have time" and "I'm not hungry."

If your problem is a lack of time, opt for convenience. Plan breakfast menus ahead, keeping them simple, yet interesting and quick to fix. Prepare for breakfast the night before or have ready-to-eat meals. For

A GOOD BREAKFAST . . .

. . . avoids highly refined breakfast cereals, which are full of added sugars and hydrogenated oils (trans fats), and includes a balance of protein, carbohydrates, and fat, appreciable amounts of essential vitamins and minerals, and food from a variety of food groups, like the following combinations:

- Cereal mix, yogurt and sliced apple, banana, and berries
- Scrambled egg, whole wheat toast, and orange sections
- Whole-grain pancakes or waffles topped with berries and yogurt, or milk
- Banana pancakes topped with fresh sliced banana, nuts, toasted oat bran, and yogurt
- String cheese, Ak-Mak crackers, apricots
- Cheese, toast, fruit
- Low-fat cream cheese on raisin bread, calcium-fortified orange juice, or milk
- Peanut butter and banana slices on a whole-grain English muffin or waffle
- Fruit smoothie with bran added and a whole-grain English muffin
- Oatmeal mixed with oat bran, nuts, low-fat milk, and a fruit or calcium-fortified orange juice

example, put the cereal bowl, spoon, and box on the kitchen counter in the evening. Then all you have to do in the morning is pour the milk.

Be a breakfast blender. Make a smoothie. Throw in some yogurt, raw nuts, and slices of your favorite fruit. Be creative.

Be untraditional. Eat a peanut butter and jelly sandwich or a turkey sandwich in the morning. Eat beans and rice wrapped in a whole wheat tortilla. Or have leftovers from the night before. Vary foods from day to day to create appetite and enthusiasm for the first meal of the day.

If your excuse is lack of hunger in the morning, take a look at the volume of food you eat after 6 P.M. Late-night eating keeps you from being hungry upon awakening. Have a light supper and no snacks so that you are hungry when you wake up in the morning. The good news is, a good breakfast makes you less hungry later in the day, so once you get into the rhythm, having a light supper comes naturally. If you're not up to a completely balanced breakfast, start gradually. Remember, something is better than nothing.

3. Unhealthy Snacking

For many people, snacking is an exercise in overindulgence and loss of control.

Healthy snacking, however, can be a great way to reduce calorie intake and get you through those edgy moments when you're starting to feel a little hungry but your next meal is still a ways off. Snacking can make you less likely to overeat at the next meal.

There's a world of healthy snacks out there. You can easily avoid junk food. Here is a sampling:

- High-fiber, high-protein cereal with fruit and milk
- High-fiber crackers and low-fat cheese
- Granola
- Tortillas: spread with light cream cheese and layered with sliced turkey, chicken, ham, or fruit, then rolled.
- Celery with peanut butter
- Broccoli, celery, and carrot sticks with light ranch dressing mixed with plain yogurt

- Jicama and cucumber slices or grape tomatoes with light ranch dressing
- Apples and light cheddar cheese
- Peaches, figs, or berries with yogurt or kefir
- Raisins and nuts or seeds (try soy nuts)
- Dried fruits with light cheese
- A handful of nuts (almonds, walnuts, cashews, pecans)

4. Dining Out and Not Watching Out

We all love to eat out. It's an occasion to sample new flavors and foods as well as to celebrate and socialize. It is also a golden opportunity to overindulge. Many people eat out more than they eat in, and this lifestyle can contribute to an excess of calories, fat, and pounds.

When dining out, avoid:

- Foods high in fat (e.g., prime rib).
- Foods prepared with added fat (e.g., hollandaise sauce).
- Restaurants with few healthy food options.
- Unnecessary waiting. When you wait, you tend to gobble up the warm white bread and butter put on the table.

Portions in restaurants are often huge, almost double the size of what we should eat. Practice portion control. Split an entrée with your companion or take half of an entrée home and eat it for lunch the next day. Fight off the temptation to indulge in all the extras: warm melt-in-your-mouth breads before the meal comes, yummy appetizers, and mouthwatering desserts. Bigger is not always better unless it's a salad with all the right stuff added (veggies, dark leafy greens, and low-fat dressing or a tasty dressing you can make right at the table with olive oil and lemon wedges).

Instead of opening up a menu and asking, "What looks good?" ask yourself "What should I eat?" A simple salad might do the trick, or a large plate filled with dark green vegetables and some feta cheese, topped with a piece of fruit.

Instead of settling for a preset item on the menu, create your own meal. Scan the menu for the foods missing from your daily intake, then piece together your entrée. For instance, order a large salad with one ounce of feta cheese and three ounces of grilled salmon on top with salad dressing on the side.

5. Overdoing the Sweet Stuff

There is no reason to deprive yourself. Life should be filled with extras that can be savored—but for your own good health, please only do it occasionally. Instead of filling your day with empty calories from foods that provide little benefit to your health, make your extras a special occasion. Eat them less often, but when you do, take the time to savor every delicious mouthful, to truly taste the food. This way, sweets become part of a celebration of a healthy life!

Remember, healthy eating consists of variety, balance, and *moderation*. Sometimes, just a taste or two of a sweet dessert is enough to satisfy the sweet tooth. Share the rest with others at the table.

Commonsense Supplementation

Many supplements have been proven to be beneficial in the pursuit of health and the treatment of illness. Without guidance from a nutritionally savvy health professional, however, people often use supplements inappropriately. They will eat a poor diet most of the time and then take a handful of supplements in the belief it will compensate and make everything okay. It's not okay. Supplements aren't replacements for eating well. They can, as the name implies, *supplement* a good diet. As such they can make up for specific nutritional shortfalls or be used in a targeted fashion—for instance, glucosamine for someone who has joint pain.

For specific applications and dosages of supplements, you should consult a knowledgeable professional. For general usage to support an active lifestyle, here are some supplement basics:

- The foundation for a good supplement program is a high-quality multivitamin and mineral formula. You can buy one in a health food store. Among the many other nutrients in the formula, it should contain the following amounts of these important factors: vitamin B_6, 400 mcg.; folic acid, 400 mcg.; vitamin C, 1,000 mg.; vitamin D, 800 international units (IU); vitamin E, 400 IU in the form of natural d-alpha tocopherol.

If you can't get a multi with these specific doses, purchase one that comes as close as possible.

- Second, take 1,000 mg. of a fish oil supplement daily. Fish oil provides important omega-3 fatty acids, which help maintain healthy blood, arteries, and heart rhythm, reduce mild hypertension and depression, and improve blood sugar metabolism and the quality of the nails, hair, and skin. Omega-3s also act as a natural anti-inflammatory and may help reduce arthritic symptoms.

  The body requires a balance of omega-6 and omega-3 fatty acids for optimum health, but the standard U.S. diet contains an extremely unhealthy overload of omega-6 fats, primarily due to excessive use of vegetable oils such as corn, canola, and sunflower. Too much omega-6 in the diet promotes inflammation in the body.

  You can increase your omega-3 intake by eating fish more often or by taking a fish oil supplement. If you burp up the fish oil, or find it otherwise unpleasant to ingest, there are refined supplements in health food stores flavored with lemon or mint that minimize the fishy taste. Using advanced technology, some food manufacturers have even started to fortify their products with micro-encapsulated fish oil. You won't taste the fish but you'll get the benefits. Foods with such fortification include breads, tortillas, milk, yogurt, and eggs. So one way or another, you shouldn't have a problem getting enough of this essential fatty acid into your diet.

- Take your supplements with a meal. That way the nutrients in the supplement are processed like food. It's best to take them earlier in the day, with breakfast or lunch.

- Don't forget adequate hydration. Drink enough liquids throughout the day, eight glasses if you can remember, and at least half of that in the form of water. Try to avoid beverages with added sugars.

- Products made from whey (a milk protein) have specific immune-supporting nutrients; and soy, egg, and casein-based products are also good.

- Individuals who are strict vegetarians or who experiment with a vegetarian diet should examine their diets carefully for adequate protein and perhaps consider the use of a protein supplement.

There's no benefit from taking a high-powered sports supplement unless you are involved in very heavy training. Then the concept becomes more valid. The extra macronutrients those products contain—carbohydrates and protein—may benefit the recovery process. *Recovery* means restoring energy to continue exercising hard the next day and rebuilding muscle tissue that has been broken down by the previous workout. In such cases, recovery requires giving the body adequate rest as well as replenishing the depleted macronutrients.

Ideally, one should replace these nutrients by having a meal within a few hours of a heavy workout. They are absorbed, utilized, and stored better by the body during this window of time. A meal as simple as a serving of rice or whole wheat bread, two vegetables, and 3 to 4 ounces of meat will fill these nutrient needs. You may not have time for a nourishing breakfast after a morning workout, however, and otherwise might be tempted to eat a bagel by itself or pick up a doughnut and a cup of coffee. For convenience and if good food is not immediately available, premixed sports supplement beverages containing protein and carbohydrates are an acceptable way to quickly replenish nutrients.

Move Yourself
Plan C

Waist Removal and Weight Loss

Plan C is about calories. If you want to trim your waist and lose weight permanently, you must burn a lot more calories with exercise and reduce your calorie intake through diet.

The success of this plan is based on hard work and resolve. You should commit to it only if you have reached the end point of the Plan B fitness programs. That means you are exercising at least five days a week. It also means you have begun to adopt a more disciplined approach to your eating habits.

If you are not exercising at least five days a week, you are not ready for Plan C. And certainly, if you are presently sedentary and have not exercised for many years, don't start here. Launching yourself into a rigorous exercise program would be foolhardy. You could easily harm yourself. Go back to Plan A.

If your goal is to move yourself to additional weight loss and waist removal, Plan C will get you there. It will improve your health and fitness while significantly reducing your risk factors for disease. And it will make you feel great!

13

Real People, Serious Results

The only way to get that fat off is to eat less and exercise more.
—Jack LaLanne

Mukidah's Transformation

For ten years, Mukidah had worked for a big telecommunications company. But in 2001 she was laid off from her project manager job along with six thousand other employees.

She was fifty-four, and like many people who are suddenly terminated, she wondered, "Now what?" She hadn't a clue what she was going to do.

On the job, she had sat in front of a computer screen much of the day and attended meetings. At home, now that her two grown-up daughters had moved on, she was far less involved in homemaking than she had been in earlier years.

She became totally sedentary, and never really thought of exercise. She owned a set of golf clubs, but played rarely, and then more for the camaraderie of friends than for the challenge of the game.

"I operated in the sluggish mode," she told us. "I could never count on having energy and I could sleep quite a lot if left alone."

Mukidah took medication for high blood pressure and, at five-feet-four and nearly 180 pounds, was extremely overweight but ignored it.

Soon after she was laid off, a friend told her about a fitness research project with sedentary postmenopausal women at our center. The friend was a personal trainer who had been nagging Mukidah for years to start exercising. She had always put her friend off.

Having nothing immediate to do, Mukidah signed up to participate in the study. The research would be going on for several years. She committed for an initial eight-month phase of the study.

The participants were randomly assigned either to do nothing or to exercise on stationary bikes and treadmills for various lengths of time. Those in the activity groups could go at their own speed, which was usually very slow. It was not an exercise program, but an experiment to collect data and see if different levels of physical activity had significant medical effects on postmenopausal women, and if so how much of an effect.

Mukidah was randomly assigned to a maximum activity group that came for nearly an hour, three or four times a week. When she was traveling or otherwise couldn't come to the center, she would put on a step counter and log her daily step total for inclusion in the study data.

"The intensity was low, just a slow speed that I could handle, with my heart rate at a certain level, and even at that I was sometimes panting," she recalled. "In the beginning, I couldn't have gone faster if I tried. And in fact, I had a hard time finishing the full amount of time I was supposed to do.

"But that changed. Within weeks I felt my energy level rising, and I felt I could go faster. The change was really exciting. I could feel my body responding. By the middle of the study, my day-in-and-day-out fatigue was gone. I could feel the growing fitness within me."

By the end of the study, the changes she saw and felt in her body had created "such a high" that she vowed never to allow herself to return to her previous sedentary state. She made physical activity a priority in her life, and continued exercising on her own.

By 2006 her weight had dropped to 147 pounds, the first time in many years she weighed below 150. She used to wear dress size twelve to fourteen. Today she wears a six or eight, and most people think she weighs around 120.

"My waist is definitely smaller," she said. "My regular pant belt was cut down and additional holes punched. I'm currently on the last hole.

"I used to avoid standing on a scale because the experience was always depressing for me," she recalled. "Not anymore."

Physical activity improved her blood pressure and cholesterol. Eventually she was able to decrease her medication to minimum dosage.

Mukidah also became disciplined with her diet. She eats much smaller portions, usually on a smaller plate. When she eats out, she gets a to-go box and immediately transfers half to two-thirds of her serving to the box, to be eaten as a meal later in the day.

Key lime pie is her favorite dessert, and "my weakness," she admitted. But only on weekends. "If I get to Sunday and have not had any dessert, I wait until the next weekend to indulge," she said. "I'm not a chocolate, candy, or cookies person. However, I do love Blue Bell ice cream. I only buy it, though, when it's on sale, and that's about once every two or three months."

Mukidah said she has had a complete about-face. "My body has not just shed pounds, and fat where I needed to lose it, but has taken a whole new well-toned shape. I've never been an athletic person but now, with lots of energy, I have developed an addiction for golf. Not only do I walk eighteen holes, but I carry my own clubs.

"I'm sixty-one years old but never felt so good. My son-in-law recently said to my daughter, 'If you're going to look like your mother when you get to her age, I'm in good shape.'"

Besides the dramatic improvement of her personal health and everyday quality of life, Mukidah's new lifestyle also produced another dividend: employment. After the original study was over, she was hired part-time at our fitness center. Today she is the center's director of member services.

She told us she purchased a pair of pants, 34 inches by 30 inches, when she started working at the center in January 2002. At the end of 2006 she gave the pants away. "To say these pants were really, really big on me would be an understatement."

Life is strange. Sometimes a bad turn of events is really a blessing in disguise.

Norm's Downsize

Like many young Oklahomans, Norm saw a future for himself in the oil and gas industry. He earned a degree in petroleum engineering, got a job in the industry, and poured himself into his work. By his early thirties, he had built a successful business and had a growing family. He was very proud about his accomplishments in life.

Along the way, however, he ignored his health. He was sedentary and overindulged in things like chicken fried steak, fried pies, ice cream, and candy. As a result, Norm ballooned to 100 pounds beyond his high school weight. He had no energy throughout the day, and by the time he got home he wanted to do nothing but vegetate in front of the television or sit in his favorite recliner and read. On those rare days when he did have some energy, he was limited physically because of pain. His back bothered him just from stooping down. His knees ached if he had to stand too long.

Norm began to realize that, just as his business success was self-made, his woeful physical condition was also of his own making. This realization led to another problem: depression. His self-image had taken a big hit.

Norm took a first baby step toward health in 1986 when he came to our clinic for a thorough physical. He was 5 feet 11 inches tall, 245 pounds, with a 44-inch waist. His fitness level was abysmal. On the exercise treadmill he tested "very poor" for cardiovascular fitness, in the bottom 20 percent of fitness. His cholesterol profile was abnormal and his blood pressure was elevated, to name just a few of the negatives. Lack of activity and poor diet were already ruining his present life and would likely shorten his life span as well.

Sometimes things have to get really bad before they get better, and in Norm's case the bad news sparked a fire inside. He returned to Oklahoma with a full head of steam to turn around his life.

He changed his eating habits the day he arrived back home. He stopped the repeat servings of fatty and sugary foods. Quality became more important than quantity. He didn't jump on a fad diet plan from some book. With the help of our nutrition staff, he had identified the undesirable elements in his diet, and now he started limiting them.

At the same time, he put activity into his life. At first it was as minimal as anyone can do: a short daily walk at a slow, steady pace. Gradually he lengthened the distance, and within the first few months he began seeing some weight loss and feeling his energy increase.

Buoyed by his improved quality of life, Norm went from slow walking to slow jogging, and then to slow long-distance running, the equivalent of a 10-minute mile.

Now in his fifties, Norm has maintained this same approach for more than twenty years. If you were to look at his medical and fitness history, as we do when he comes periodically for checkups, you would think you were dealing with a totally different person.

Norm weighs 165 pounds and measures 31 inches at the waist. On the treadmill, he consistently scores in the "superior" fitness category. He's a man enjoying life in a way that was impossible for him when he was younger. He's full of energy and free of pain. The depression disappeared long ago, soon after he resumed activity and learned how to balance his life so he can enjoy all of it—business, family, and personal health. The balance includes an occasional reward of a combo chocolate-raspberry ice cream double scoop—his favorite flavors—which he relishes without a single tug of guilt.

We see cases like Mukidah's and Norm's all the time at our center. And every once in a while we have monster successes like Gina, an obese twenty-six-year-old schoolteacher who entered our weight loss program in 2002. She was as sedentary as they come. She checked in at 5 feet 3 inches and 340 pounds.

A typical day for her was to get up, eat, get in the car and drive to work, walk to the classroom, eat lunch, return to the classroom, get in the car, and drive home or go to a fast-food restaurant for dinner, watch TV, and go to sleep.

Gina started our program with a step counter and with the instructions to add up to 500 daily steps each week. Today she runs in 5K and 10K races. She's far from the fastest, but she is out there running. She didn't follow a specific diet plan; she just switched from full-sized fast-food meals to kiddie portions. That worked for her, and accommodated her lifestyle habit of eating out a lot.

Gina got herself down to 176 pounds—still overweight—but she has much better health and her risks for disease are greatly reduced. Plus, she feels a whole better and enjoys life much more.

Gina, at half her previous body weight, is a shining example of how reasonable, manageable physical activity and dietary changes that fit into one's lifestyle are the changes that stick.

Watch Your Belly Fat

For patients with weight issues, unless we are dealing with an egregious obesity problem, we tend to first emphasize neutralizing excess belly fat and deal with weight loss second. As we discussed earlier, men with a waist size greater than 40 inches and women with a waist size greater than 35 inches literally house a toxin factory within. The inflammatory substances spewed out by this midsection fat zone eat away at health, molecule by molecule. Excess belly fat is the trademark of the metabolic syndrome, a gateway to life-threatening physical disorders.

At our center, we first measure the waist circumference to identify patients who need to lose weight. Then we recommend using the scale as a behavioral tool to achieve a specific waist and weight goal. Here's what we mean: if you are over the waist size limit, you should lose 10 percent of your weight in one year. That's a reasonable and realistic goal.

Your waist and your weight go hand in hand. Two sides of the same coin.

As we have pointed out throughout the book, there are tremendous quality-of-life and health benefits generated by physical activity. Independently, there are many quality-of-life and health benefits generated by waist and weight loss, even if after the 10 percent weight loss you still have not reached a normal weight level, or your waist circumference has not shrunk significantly.

Usually a 10 percent weight loss comes with some waist shrinkage. With that kind of weight loss, you'll probably rid yourself of 30 to 40 percent of your dangerous visceral adiposity. So the weight you lose includes toxic weight—the visceral fat. You use the scale not to bring you down to some artificial number but to conveniently and meaningfully track the loss of the belly fat. So be more concerned about trimming your waist than your weight. By downsizing your belly fat, you neutralize the toxin factory.

The heavier you are, the more important is the 10 percent loss. Forget about losing 50 or 75 pounds. Your body will be very thankful for a 10 percent loss over a year.

Plan C will do the job for you. It will improve your health, and in the process usually will improve your metabolic syndrome risk factor numbers (waist circumference, blood pressure, blood sugar, HDL, and triglycerides).

From our observation with patients, thirty days into this program your dresses or pants should fit much looser. The tape measure will tell you how much circumference you have lost. If your waist was 42 inches, it should now be 41 or 40 inches. Man or woman, within the first few weeks you should see some waist removal and weight loss.

Even though we haven't done actual studies on waist-size shrink-age, our observation has been that the shrinkage will eventually slow down. Regarding weight loss, we find that people who go on this pro-gram often lose 6 to 8 pounds in thirty days. That's a desirable rate of reduction.

What if you are the exception and don't lose weight or reduce your waist, or you lose just a little? Should you get frustrated? Absolutely not. Remember that physical activity alone, even at the level of Plan A, reduces the ability of visceral fat to poison your body. That's extremely reassuring.

Beyond that, ask yourself how you feel. How's your heartburn? Your constipation? Your fatigue? Your sex drive? Or any quality-of-life issues important to you? If you feel better, that's a magnificent result. Just stay with the program. Waist removal and weight loss are like icing on the cake.

The Five Keys to Successful Waist Removal and Weight Loss

Most anybody can lose weight. Keeping it off is the challenge, and it's almost impossible without physical activity. Research, including ours, shows that you have just about a zero chance to keep weight off by diet alone. Unfortunately, the focus in this country has been on dieting and weight loss instead of on healthy behavior.

Diets come and diets go. Beyond all the hoopla and best-sellers, no-nonsense nutritionists and dietitians still resort to the basic rule of thumb for weight loss: calories in, calories out. If you want to trim your waist and lose weight permanently, you must exercise more (increase the calories you burn) and eat less (reduce the calories you take in).

We've seen thousands of patients try to lose paunches and weight over the years. Based on the current research and on our experience we find that the ones who take it off—and keep it off—do the following five things consistently:

1. Exercise.

2. Reduce the calories they eat.

3. Eat breakfast.

4. Log, log, log, log.

    Logging keeps you tuned in to the process. Makes you pay attention. Makes you accountable day by day. Without logging there is a real tendency to overestimate your energy expenditure and underestimate your consumption. It's just human nature. Log anything and everything that you regard as important to help you reach your goal, such as steps, minutes of activity, your daily weight, and daily intake of fat grams and total calories. It's up to you. At a minimum, track your activity, diet, and weight. The more variables you include, the more likely will be your success at losing and keeping weight off.

5. Take it slow and steady.

    You are not in a race. The American mentality is to want to be the hare. To get fast results. A quick fix. But when it comes to behavioral changes that modify your life, you want to be like the tortoise. Slow and steady wins in the end. That is an essential—but typically overlooked—element in any kind of weight-loss program. The faster you lose weight, the faster you are likely to put it back on. You cannot view weight loss as a short-term project. It has to become a long-term lifestyle habit. Your goal is to adopt lifelong behaviors that will create and sustain a maximally healthy constitution, weight, and figure.

14

Move Yourself
Five Days a Week

Move more. Lose more.

—Anonymous

I f you have reached the end point of any of the Plan B activity programs, you are at the door of Plan C. If you have not reached that
level, if you are not exercising at least five days a week, go back to chapter 4 and assess where your starting point should be. Be patient, and take
our program step by step. Plan A and Plan B both will bring you solid
health benefits; Plan B will prepare you to go on to Plan C, the next step
up for weight and belly-fat loss.

The five-day frequency factor is important for weight loss and calorie burning. Let's say you go out and walk briskly for 45 minutes. You
rev up your metabolism, and your body doesn't immediately return to its
pre-exercise state. Just as in a car, the engine is still hot, so to speak.
Over the next few hours your system cools down, and during that "trail-
off" period you are burning calories at an accelerated rate. So by
increasing the frequency of exercise—to five days or more per week—
you collect more of those "trail-off" times.

To FIT and Beyond

For effective waist removal and to lose that 10 percent of weight, you must now go beyond the FIT formula in Plan B, and do the following:

- First, remember the frequency (the F factor) of your workouts—it must be maintained at five times a week.
- Now, increase the time (the T factor) up to 45-plus minutes a session. Build up the T factor over a month.
- Once you have F and T where you want them, start increasing the I factor—intensity.

Use the sample chart below for a basic guide. The cardio routines that follow provide more specifics as you advance in the program.

FREQUENCY

	Week 1	Week 2	Week 3	Week 4
Aerobics		Monday–Friday		
Strength		Tuesday, Thursday		
Stretching		Most days		

Try to get in aerobic activity every day if possible. If you are unable to amass enough aerobic minutes during the week, try to make up for it on weekends with a long walk, hike, or bike ride. For many people, Saturday mornings offer a good opportunity to accumulate a lot of activity.

INTENSITY

	Week 1	Week 2	Week 3	Week 4
Aerobics	Moderate, slightly heavy breathing but able to converse in short sentences			
Strength		12–15 repetitions per set		
Stretching		30 seconds per set		

TIME

	Week 1	Week 2	Week 3	Week 4
Aerobics	30 minutes	35 minutes	40 minutes	45 minutes
Strength		2 sets each exercise		
Stretching		30 seconds per stretch		

Waist Removal and Weight Loss Cardio Programs

WALKING

Week	Distance (miles)	Time (minutes)	Frequency/Week (times)
1	4.0	55:00	5
2	4.0	54:00	5
3	4.0	53:00	5
4	4.0	52:00	5

JOGGING

Week	Distance (miles)	Time (minutes)	Frequency/Week (times)
1	3.5	35:00	5
2	4.0	40:00	5
3	4.0	38:00	5
4	4.0	36:00	5

SWIMMING

Week	Distance (yards)	Time (minutes)	Frequency/Week (times)
1	1,400	27:00	5
2	1,800	34:30	5
3	2,000	39:00	5
4	2,400	47:30	5

CYCLING (Stationary or Outdoors)

Week	Speed (MPH)	Time (minutes)	Frequency/Week (times)
1	20	35:00	5
2	20	45:00	5
3	20	55:00	5
4	20	60:00	5

A Calorie-Burning Alternative for Joggers Who Can't Jog

You can't do much better for calorie burning than repeatedly throwing your body weight and catching it. That may sound like a strange concept. But that's what defines running or jogging, as compared to the gliding nature of walking. Both feet are off the ground at some point during each stride. This repeated throwing and catching of body weight takes more effort and burns more calories.

However, we don't recommend jogging for everybody, particularly individuals with a history of ankle, knee, hip, back, or neck problems. Jogging involves a significantly bigger impact on your weight-bearing joints than walking does. It's better for calorie burning, but harder on you orthopedically.

Consider power-walking as an alternative. In Plan B (chapter 8) we related the story of Casey Meyers, the runner who turned to power-walking after two knee surgeries. He found that by revving up his walking speed, he could achieve as good a calorie burn as jogging.

How fast is power-walking? Picture the days years ago when you splashed around in a public or community swimming pool crowded with kids. Posted signs abound in such places: do not run. Yet kids are kids, and tend to ignore the warning. They'll run anyway on the wet and slippery decks, typically evoking a loud warning from the lifeguard to slow down and walk.

So what happens? Kids will gear down into an erect, arms-a-pumping, legs-a-churning power-walk. They're still in a hurry. They're going about as fast as they can go without actually running. That's power-walking. Try it if you are joint-challenged. It certainly is a joint-friendly way to go.

You may think that a power walk can't match the calorie expenditure of jogging. But you'd be wrong. It's like a car with a manual transmission running in a low gear. The engine (and you) operate more efficiently once you get up to speed and shift into a higher gear, but at a low gear you burn more fuel.

At some point, as you stick with the program, you will reach your target weight. When that happens give yourself a huge pat on the back and celebrate the accomplishment. But you can't say, "Hurray for me, I did it," and then stop the program. That's a ticket for putting the weight right back on.

Now it's a matter of long-term weight maintenance. That means assessing your program—both the activity and the diet that we lay out in the next chapter—and following it month after month to the degree you need in order to maintain your target weight. You'll have to experiment with it to see what works best for you.

15

Move Yourself Plan C Diet and Supplements

My doctor told me to stop having intimate dinners for four. Unless there are three other people.

—Orson Welles

From 1979 to 2004, Georgia Kostas, M.P.H., R.D., served as director of nutrition at our center. During that time she counseled some twenty-five thousand individuals on how to eat right, and for many overweight patients she prescribed calorie-restrictive diets as part of a comprehensive lifestyle program. Today she has her own nutritional consulting firm in Dallas (www.georgiakostas.com).

Georgia was kind enough to share her experience with us in the form of eating tips and two reduced-calorie menus—a 1,300-calorie diet for women, and a 1,600-calorie diet for men. We use these guidelines for our Plan C eating program. The nutritionally balanced menus have been computer-analyzed to ensure they meet 100 percent of all recommended nutrient needs, even while reducing calories.

Before You Start—
Tips for Success

One of the best ways to stick to a diet is to write down everything you eat. Log your meals before eating them. Listing specific amounts of food consumed is ideal, but it even works if you just identify "small" portion of this, or "large" portion of that. You may not think this could be an effective measure, but it is very helpful. Writing before eating implies making a conscious decision about what you are going to eat. This mindfulness can make a big difference between eating three cookies or eating ten.

One patient has been logging her meals and her exercise for twenty-four years without missing a day. You might think such behavior obsessive, but she has been able to keep weight off for all that time. For someone under 5 feet tall, weight was always a challenge for her. She originally wanted to lose 20 pounds for her twentieth high school reunion. That's like a 6-footer trying to lose 50 pounds. Recording her meals and activity worked so well for that short-term goal that she made it a goal for the long term—the rest of her life.

Another helpful habit to get into is to eat foods that are less calorie-dense. You can eat more of these foods, which will make you feel full. You need to get a feeling of satisfaction and fullness from the calories you eat. Some people can't stick to a reduced-calorie diet because they eat small volumes of food for those calories. For instance, you might not feel as full from a 100-calorie slice of cheese as you would from a 100-calorie serving of Cheerios (1.5 cups) or popcorn (4 cups).

It also really helps you reach or maintain your weight goal if you can redistribute your calories throughout the day, meaning that you eat more at breakfast and lunch, and eat less at dinner. For instance, consume 75 percent of your calories during the day and only 25 percent at dinner. You may not find it practical all the time, but give it a try and see how it might work for you.

This is the opposite of how we usually eat in our society. People often rush out the door in the morning, skip breakfast or grab something not so wholesome to eat on the run, eat a fast lunch, and then pile it on later in the day, beginning with snacks and drinks, a heavy meal, dessert, and more snacks after dinner.

This pattern of eating heavily late in the day is one of the biggest obstacles to weight loss. Evening is when you are the most sedentary, and the excess calories go to fat more readily. Of course, it's different if you go dancing in the evening. You would be burning off some of the evening calories.

Eating more during your active daytime hours will allow you to eat more overall and still lose weight. Calorie reversal in this manner is effective, but we have found it impractical for many people who eat their dinners in a social setting—either at home with family, or out with friends—where they generally like to be able to eat more. For this reason, we eventually stopped recommending it, but not before we did some research with patients. We indeed found that those who could pull it off—eating most of their calories during the day instead of at night—were able to lose more weight. If you can, make your dinner your lunch, and make your lunch or breakfast your dinner. If you can't, don't worry about it. Just eat mindfully.

Expect progress, but not perfection, when you make dietary changes.

It also helps to have a particular pattern of eating at meals. For example, routinely include a fruit with breakfast, lunch, and snack, or regularly have two or three servings of vegetables at supper. Patterns build consistency, making balanced eating easier.

Finally, be aware of when you are full. You don't have to finish what is in front of you. If a meal is too big, save part of it for a later snack.

Consider the plan as a guide that you try to follow as closely as you can without letting it become stressful. That would defeat the purpose of improving your health. Nobody sticks to rigid menus perfectly anyway. Some people may repeat a favored daily menu selection several times a week. Whatever your changes are, do make an effort to stay within the number of daily servings for each food group, but within each group feel free to substitute. Some foods obviously will be more to your liking and others are more convenient to prepare.

When you reach your goal, what next? Gradually increase your portions or add back food that you miss the most. You'll have to experiment so that you don't start gaining weight back. Try to stay within a range of 500 additional calories, and ideally limit yourself to 200 or 300 more. That will give you the leeway for fun foods here and there, such as a piece of cake at a family or office celebration or a glass of wine for dinner. If you are a woman, check out the 1,600-calorie diet for men. That's a good plan to follow once you reach your goal with the 1,300-calorie diet.

Georgia Kostas's
Reduced-Calorie Diet

The pages that follow contain a fourteen-day program of reduced-calorie menus for women, followed by fourteen days of menus for men.

You can trade items within each daily menu. For instance, substitute an apple with another snack instead of a dessert for lunch. As mentioned earlier, have your larger meal earlier in the day if you can. Keep in mind that each daily menu was designed to give you 100 percent of your nutritional needs for the day.

Within this plan, it's quite acceptable to substitute food that you prefer, but stay within a food group, meaning switch one type of meat for another, one vegetable for another vegetable.

Drink an 8 to 12 ounce glass of water with every meal, and 36 additional ounces of water throughout the day.

You may add three "extra" foods a week, up to 100 to 150 calories each, such as:

- ½ cup (4 oz.) frozen fat-free, sugar-free yogurt or ice milk (80 to 110 calories)
- ½ cup (4 oz.) fat-free chocolate pudding snack (Jell-O, Hunt's, etc.) (100 calories)
- 1 low-calorie frozen ice cream treat (80 to 100 calories)
- 5 vanilla wafers (80 calories)
- 2 fig newtons (120 calories)
- 2 tbsp. light syrup such as maple (60 calories)

About meat: When you substitute meats, be sure the replacement is lean. Instead of chicken, you may like fresh fish, or a filet mignon or sirloin. A lean pork chop will work, but not a fatty rib.

About milk: Soy milk may be substituted for regular milk in any menus. Choose fat-free, fortified with calcium. Soy yogurt and low-fat cheese may also be substituted.

About cheese: Note that in the daily menus cheese has been counted as either a milk-dairy or meat/protein item. Cheese is unique in its ability to be included in either category.

Vegetarians: Trade a 2 oz. meat portion for ½ cup beans or tofu, or 1 oz. low-fat cheese; and trade a 3 oz. meat portion for ¾ cup beans or tofu, or 1½ oz. low-fat cheese.

About fats: Feel free to choose lower-fat versions of cheese, dressings, mayonnaise, and so on, in the menus.

Light dressings refer to those averaging 25 calories per tablespoon. Read labels. They can range from 15 to 50 calories per tablespoon.

You may use butter flavorings (e.g., I Can't Believe It's Not Butter spray) and nonstick vegetable oil cooking sprays whenever desired. If you prefer to use less fat than the menu suggests, go ahead. You'll save 50 calories per fat serving.

About vegetables: If you can eat more vegetables per menu, add them. Never skimp on veggies! Eat as many as you can.

Other ideas: grill or roast veggies (eggplant, broccoli, red bell pepper, etc.), steam fresh celery and carrots, or blend frozen vegetables, such as 1 package of broccoli with cheese sauce, or 1 package of spinach with 1 package of creamed or buttered spinach. And don't forget to try sugar-snap beans (fresh or frozen)—everyone's favorite!

Try edamame beans (these are a type of soybean eaten right out of the pods). Just steam a frozen bag for 5 minutes and eat as finger food. Eat 1 bag (16 oz.) and count it as 4 vegetables—sweet and delicious and fun to eat!

About breads and grains: Note these bread (starch) substitutes: 2 toasts = 1 English muffin = 1 small bagel (e.g., Lender's) = ½ deli bagel. You can substitute grits, oatmeal, hot cereal/grains for cold cereals in the menus, or let cereal replace bread (2 toasts = 1 cup cereal).

Choose whole grains first.

About seasonings: Add salsa, cilantro, pico de gallo, onion, garlic, bell pepper, jalapenos, spices, and herbs to give pizzazz to any menu items.

About fruits and juices: Choose calcium-fortified citrus juices (orange, grapefruit, tangerine, etc.). If you like, substitute your favorite fruits for any appearing in the menus to follow.

About color: Note the red and green food in most lunch and dinner menus—the colors are signs of super-nutrition!

Shopping Tips

- Buy pantry items in the smallest available packages.
- Shop at stores with salad bars or precut fruits and vegetables for your convenience.
- Keep extra bread products, cheese, deli items, and butcher meats in the freezer until needed.
- Take advantage of the deli, butcher, and bakery departments to buy individual portions.
- Keep these condiments on hand: light cream cheese, soft tub margarine, light tub margarine (1 tbsp. = 35 to 50 calories), light or fat-free salad dressings (ranch, Italian, vinaigrette, coleslaw, Catalina), balsamic vinegar, salsa, sugar-free jam/jelly, apple butter, light (reduced-calorie) maple syrup, light or fat-free mayonnaise, mustard, olive oil, dill pickles, Knorr bouillon cubes (chicken).

Fourteen-Day Menu for Women (1,300 calories)

Each day's menu provides the following number of servings for each food group: 2 milk (*Mk*), 5 meat (*Mt*), 5 starches (*St*), 3 fruits (*Fr*), 3-plus vegetables (*Vg*), 4 fat (*Ft*).

- To make 1,200 calories: omit 2 fat servings.
- To make 1,400 calories: add 100 calories of choice as a snack, extra starch, or large fruit.
- "Free" foods in the menus are items with negligible calories, so you may eat them freely.
- After completing two weeks, return to Day 1 menu.
- In the menus, tbsp. = tablespoon, tsp. = teaspoon, c. = cup, oz. = ounce

DAY 1

Breakfast

½ c. calcium-fortified orange juice or 1 fresh orange (*1 Fr*)

1 whole wheat toast (*1 St*) with 1 tsp. sugar-free jam/jelly (*Free*) and 1½ tbsp. peanut butter or 1 tsp. tub margarine (*1 Ft*)

1 c. fat-free milk (*1 Mk*)

Lunch

tuna sandwich:

> 2 slices whole wheat bread (*2 St*)
>
> ½ c. water-packed tuna (*2 Mt*) mixed with 1 tbsp. light mayonnaise (*1 Ft*) and ¼ c. chopped apple, celery, and pickle (*Free*)
>
> lettuce and tomato slices (*Free*)

1 small apple (*1 Fr*)

1 c. fat-free milk (*1 Mk*)

Dinner

3 oz. skinless chicken breast, grilled (*3 Mt*)

1 small red (new) potato (*1 St*) with butter-flavor spray (*Free*)

½ c. carrots, steamed (*1 Vg*)

½ c. green beans, steamed (*1 Vg*)

1 c. green salad (*Free*) with 1 sliced tomato (*1 Vg*) and 2 tbsp. light dressing (*1 Ft*)

½ c. fresh pineapple chunks (*1 Fr*)

Snack

3 c. microwave light popcorn (*1 St, 1 Ft*)

DAY 2

Breakfast

   1 c. cubed or ¼ cantaloupe (*1 Fr*)

   ½ whole wheat English muffin (*1 St*) with 1 tsp. apple butter (*Free*)
      and 1½ tbsp. peanut butter or 1 tsp. tub margarine (*1 Ft*)

   1 c. fat-free milk (*1 Mk*)

Lunch

   1 small whole wheat bagel or 2 slices bread (*2 St*)

   2 oz. low-fat cheese (*2 Mt*)

   1 raw carrot, in sticks (*1 Vg*)

   1 small pear (*1 Fr*)

   1 c. fat-free, sugar-free yogurt (*1 Mk*)

Dinner

   3 oz. broiled fish with lemon (3 Mt) with 1 tsp. melted margarine (*1 Ft*)

   ½ c. corn, steamed (*1 St*)

   ½ c. Brussels sprouts, steamed (*1 Vg*)

   1 tsp. (or 1 tbsp. light) margarine for vegetables (*1 Ft*)

   1 c. romaine lettuce salad (Free) with 1 sliced tomato (*1 Vg*) and 1
      tbsp. French dressing (*1 Ft*)

   ½ c. fresh fruit salad (*1 Fr*)

Snack

   5 whole wheat low-fat Triscuit crackers

DAY 3

Breakfast

   ½ banana (*1 Fr*)

   ½ c. bran flakes or Kashi cereal (*1 St*)

   1 tbsp. almonds (*1 Ft*)

   1 c. fat-free milk (*1 Mk*)

Lunch

  turkey sandwich:

    2 slices whole wheat bread (*2 St*)

    2 oz. turkey (*2 Mt*)

    1 tbsp. light mayonnaise (*1 Ft*)

    lettuce, tomato slices (*Free*)

  1 small apple (*1 Fr*)

  1 c. fat-free milk (*1 Mk*)

Dinner

  3 oz. lean beef tenderloin (*3 Mt*)

  ½ c. brown rice (*1 St*) cooked in broth (*Free*)

  ½ c. zucchini (*1 Vg*) and ½ c. yellow squash (*1 Vg*) stir-fried in
    1 tsp. oil (*1 Ft*)

  1 spinach salad (*Free*) with 1 small tomato (*1 Vg*) and 2 tbsp. light
    dressing (*1 Ft*)

  1 orange, in sections (*1 Fr*)

Snack

  3 graham cracker squares (*1 St*)

DAY 4

Breakfast

  ½ grapefruit (*1 Fr*)

  1 small whole wheat bagel (*2 St*) with 1½ tbsp. light cream cheese
    (*1 Ft*)

  1 c. fat-free milk (*1 Mk*)

Lunch

  1 small red (new) potato (*1 St*) topped with ½ c. low-fat cottage
    cheese (*2 Mt*)

  1 large romaine lettuce salad (*Free*) with sliced cucumbers, onions,
    celery, cherry tomatoes (*Free*) with 2 tbsp. light dressing (*1 Ft*)

½ c. asparagus (*1 Vg*) sautéed in 1 tsp. oil (*1 Ft*)

1 c. strawberries (*1 Fr*)

Dinner

spaghetti:

3 oz. extra-lean ground beef, cooked and drained (*3 Mt*)

½ c. meatless spaghetti sauce (*1 St*) over ½ c. cooked spaghetti (*1 St*), 4 c. spinach (½ c. cooked) (*1 Vg*) and ½ c. mushrooms and onions (*1 Vg*) sautéed in 1 tsp. olive oil (*1 Ft*) and lemon juice

1 c. melon, cubed (*1 Fr*)

Snack

8 oz. fat-free, sugar-free lemon yogurt (*1 Mk*)

DAY 5

Breakfast

1 orange (*1 Fr*)

½ c. oatmeal, cooked (*1 St*)

1 tbsp. walnuts (*1 Ft*)

1 c. fat-free milk (*1 Mk*)

Lunch

pita turkey sandwich:

1 pita pocket (*2 St*)

2 oz. turkey (*2 Mt*)

1 oz. (2 slices) low-fat cheese (*1 Mk*)

lettuce, tomato slices (*Free*)

1 tbsp. mustard (*Free*)

1 c. grapes (*1 Fr*)

½ c. V8 or tomato juice (*1 Vg*)

Dinner

    3 oz. baked seafood (*3 Mt*)

    ½ c. mashed potatoes (*1 St*) with 1 tbsp. light margarine (*1 Ft*)

    1 c. broccoli-carrot-onion-mushroom mix (*2 Vg*), stir-fried with 1 tsp. olive oil (*1 Ft*)

    mixed green salad (Free) with 2 tbsp. light dressing (*1 Ft*)

    ½ cup fruit salad (*1 Fr*)

Snack

    2 large flavored rice cakes or 1 c. Cheerios (*1 St*)

DAY 6

Breakfast

    1 c. fat-free plain yogurt (*1 Mk*) topped with ½ banana (*1 Fr*) and ⅓ c. Kashi Go Lean Crunch cereal (*1 St*)

Lunch

    chef salad:

        2 c. mixed salad greens (*Free*) with ½ c. raw broccoli and ½ c. raw cauliflower (*1 Vg*)

        1 tomato, sliced (*1 Vg*)

        2 oz. turkey ham (*2 Mt*)

        1 oz. low-fat cheese (*1 Mt*)

        4 tbsp. light dressing (*2 Ft*)

    1 fresh peach (*1 Fr*)

    1 c. vegetable soup or 4 Rye-Krisps (*1 St*)

Dinner

    2 slices of a medium cheese pizza, thin crust (*2 Mt, 2 St, 2 Ft*)

    1 c. cucumber, onion, and tomato (*1 Vg*)

    1¼ c. watermelon (*1 Fr*)

Snack

16 oz. (2 c.) sugar-free, fat-free hot cocoa (*1 Mk*)

3 graham cracker squares or 5 low-fat Triscuit crackers (*1 St*)

DAY 7

Breakfast

½ c. calcium-fortified orange juice or ½ c. blueberries (*1 Fr*)

1 four-inch whole wheat pancake (*1 St*) with 1 tbsp. light syrup (*1 Ft*) and 1 tbsp. light margarine (*1 Ft*)

1 c. fat-free milk (*1 Mk*)

Lunch

3 oz. skinless chicken breast (*3 Mt*)

½ c. rice, cooked in chicken broth (*1 St*)

½ c. green peas, steamed (*1 St*)

½ c. carrots, steamed (*1 Vg*) with 1 tsp. margarine (*1 Ft*)

½ c. cabbage, shredded (slaw) (*Free*) with 2 tbsp. light dressing (*1 Ft*)

1 c. cubed or ¼ of a cantaloupe (*1 Fr*)

Dinner

taco salad:

½ c. pinto or kidney beans (*1 St, 1 Mt*)

1 oz. (¼ c.) low-fat cheese (*1 Mt*)

1 tomato, sliced (*1 Vg*)

1 c. chopped raw vegetables (bell pepper, carrots, red onions, etc.) (*1 Vg*)

1 c. lettuce (*Free*)

1 corn tortilla, toasted and broken into chips (*1 St*)

4 tbsp. salsa (*Free*)

½ c. fresh pineapple chunks (*1 Fr*)

Snack

1 c. fat-free, sugar-free strawberry yogurt (*1 Mk*)

DAY 8

Breakfast

1 fresh orange (*1 Fr*)

1 whole wheat English muffin (*2 St*) topped with 3 tbsp. (¼ c.) part-skim mozzarella cheese (*1 Mt*)

1 c. fat-free milk (*1 Mk*)

Lunch

fast-food grilled chicken breast sandwich (no mayonnaise) (*2 St, 3 Mt*)

1 small apple (*1 Fr*)

1 c. fat-free milk (*1 Mk*) (or occasional 4 oz. fat-free, sugar-free frozen yogurt)

Dinner

vegetarian stir-fry:

Heat in skillet in 3 tsp. oil, (*3 Ft*): 1½ c. mixed vegetables (*3 Vg*), ½ c. onions and mushrooms (*1 Vg*)

½ c. steamed brown rice (*1 St*)

½ c. fresh pineapple chunks (*1 Fr*) with ¼ c. low-fat cottage cheese (*1 Mt*)

1 fortune cookie (*Free*)

Snack

1 wedge/slice of low-fat cheese (*1 Mk*)

DAY 9

Breakfast

¼ cantaloupe (*1 Fr*)

1 cinnamon-raisin bagel (*2 St*) with 1½ tbsp. light cream cheese (*1 Ft*)

8 oz. fat-free, sugar-free peach yogurt (*1 Mk*)

Lunch

1 c. lentil or bean soup (*1 St, 1 Vg, 1 Mt*)

1 c. tossed green salad (*Free*) with 1 (or 2 tbsp. light) ranch dressing (*1 Ft*) and 3 tbsp. Parmesan cheese (*1 Mt*) and 1 tbsp. walnuts (*1 Ft*)

½ c. fresh fruit salad (*1 Fr*)

Dinner

3 oz. turkey or skinless chicken breast, roasted (*3 Mt*)

½ c. corn, steamed (*1 St*)

½ c. carrots, steamed (*1 Vg*)

4 c. raw spinach (½ c. cooked) (*1 Vg*) sautéed in 1 tsp. olive oil (*1 Ft*)

15-calorie sugar-free popsicle (*Free*)

Snack

1 c. fat-free milk (*1 Mk*)

1 c. grapes (*1 Fr*)

DAY 10

Breakfast

1 banana (*2 Fr*)

1 c. shredded wheat (*2 St*)

1 tbsp. chopped nuts (*1 Ft*)

1 c. fat-free milk (*1 Mk*)

Lunch

soft tacos:

2 corn tortillas (*2 St*), 2 oz. skinless chicken (*2 Mt*), ¼ c. low-fat cheese, grated (*1 Mk*), ¼ tomato, diced (*Free*), shredded lettuce (*Free*), and 3 tbsp. salsa (*Free*)

1 fresh peach (*1 Fr*)

Dinner

3 oz. red snapper (*3 Mt*) sautéed in 2 tsp. oil (*2 Ft*)

½ c. red (new) potatoes, grilled (*1 St*)

½ c. yellow squash, grilled (*1 Vg*)

½ c. zucchini, grilled (*1 Vg*)

1 tsp. olive oil, for grilling vegetables (*1 Ft*), and 2 tbsp. balsamic vinegar (*Free*)

1 fresh tomato, in wedges (*1 Vg*)

DAY 11

Breakfast

1 c. fresh strawberries (*1 Fr*)

⅓ c. Kashi Go Lean Crunch cereal (*1 St*) and 1 tbsp. nuts (*1 Ft*) on top of 8 oz. plain, fat-free yogurt (*1 Mk*)

Lunch

tuna sandwich:

2 slices light whole wheat bread (*1 St*)

½ c. water-packed tuna (*2 Mt*), mixed with 1 tbsp. light mayonnaise (*1 Ft*) and 3 tbsp. chopped celery, apple, and pickle (*Free*)

lettuce and tomato slices (*Free*)

1 fresh small pear or apple (*1 Fr*)

Dinner

low-calorie frozen dinner (up to 300 cal., 10 g fat) (*3 Mt, 1 St, 1 Vg*)

½ c. broccoli, steamed (*1 Vg*), with 1 tbsp. slivered almonds (*1 Ft*) and 1 tsp. margarine (*1 Ft*)

½ c. carrots, steamed (*1 Vg*)

1 whole wheat roll or bread slice (*1 St*) with butter-flavor spray (*Free*)

Snack

1 c. fat-free milk (*1 Mk*)

1 c. grapes (*1 Fr*)

3 graham cracker squares (*1 St*)

DAY 12

Breakfast

½ grapefruit (*1 Fr*)

1 fat-free Eggo or Kashi waffle (*1 St*) with 1 tbsp. light syrup (*1 Ft*) and 1 tbsp. light margarine (*1 Ft*)

8 oz. fat-free, sugar-free strawberry yogurt or 1 c. fat-free milk (*1 Mk*)

Lunch

hamburger:

1 bun (*2 St*), 3 oz. 90% lean ground beef (*3 Mt*)

1 slice low-fat cheddar cheese (50 cal./oz.) (*1 Mt*)

lettuce, tomato, mustard (*Free*)

1 c. watermelon slices (*1 Fr*)

1 c. fat-free milk (*1 Mk*) or occasional 4 oz. fat-free, sugar-free pudding snack

Dinner

shrimp creole:

1 oz. (5 large) boiled shrimp (*1 Mt*) heated in ½ c. spaghetti sauce (*1 St*) served over ½ c. brown rice (*1 St*)

1½ c. vegetable mix (broccoli, cauliflower, carrots, etc.) (*3 Vg*), stir-fried in 2 tsp. oil (*2 Ft*)

1 c. cantaloupe slices (¼ melon) (*1 Fr*)

Snack

1 c. fat-free milk (*1 Mk*)

1 c. grapes (*1 Fr*)

DAY 13

Breakfast

½ c. calcium-fortified orange juice or 1 fresh orange (*1 Fr*)

1 whole wheat toast (*1 St*) with 1 tsp. sugar-free jam (*Free*)

1 poached egg (*1 Mt*)

1 c. fat-free milk (*1 Mk*)

Lunch

pasta salad:

> 1 c. pasta, cooked (*2 St*), ½ c. chopped vegetables (broccoli, car-rots, onions, red bell pepper) (*1 Vg*), with 3 to 4 tbsp. light Italian dressing (*2 Ft*) and 3 tbsp. grated Parmesan cheese (*1 Mt*)

spinach salad (*Free*) with 2 tbsp. light Catalina dressing (*1 Ft*)

½ c. fresh fruit salad (*1 Fr*)

1 c. fat-free milk (*1 Mk*)

Dinner

fajitas:

> 2 soft whole wheat tortillas (*2 St*), 3 oz. grilled flank steak (*3 Mt*) marinated in 2 tbsp. lime juice (*Free*) and ½ tsp. fajita seasoning (*Free*)

> ½ c. onion and bell peppers (*1 Vg*), grilled in 1 tsp. oil (*1 Ft*)

> ½ c. tomato, diced (*1 Vg*)

> ½ c. lettuce, shredded (*Free*)

½ c. fresh pineapple chunks (*1 Fr*)

DAY 14

Breakfast

1 c. strawberries or ½ c. blueberries (*1 Fr*)

2 four-inch whole wheat pancakes (*2 St*) with 2 tbsp. light syrup (*1 Ft*)

1 c. fat-free milk or yogurt (*1 Mk*)

Lunch

3 oz. skinless chicken breast (*3 Mt*), marinated in 3 tbsp. fat-free Italian dressing (*Free*) and baked, grilled, or broiled

½ c. mashed potatoes (*1 St*) with 1 tsp. (1 tbsp. light) margarine (*1 Ft*)

½ c. cabbage, shredded (*Free*) with 1 tbsp. coleslaw dressing (*1 Ft*)

½ c. yellow squash, steamed (*1 Vg*)

½ c. green beans, steamed (*1 Vg*)

1 tbsp. light margarine (*1 Ft*)

1 c. watermelon slices (*1 Fr*)

1 c. fat-free milk (*1 Mk*)

Dinner

mini-pizzas:

> 2 whole wheat English muffin halves (*2 St*) topped with 1 oz. (3 tbsp.) grated part-skim mozzarella cheese (*3 Mt*)
>
> 1 oz. (2 slices) Canadian bacon or smoked turkey (*1 Mt*)
>
> 2 tbsp. mushrooms, sliced (*Free*)
>
> 2 tbsp. onion, diced (*Free*)
>
> 2 tbsp. green pepper, diced (*Free*)
>
> ¼ c. pizza sauce (*Free*)

1 c. raw vegetables (*1 Vg*) (carrot sticks, celery, broccoli, tomato, cucumber, etc.)

1 fresh orange, in sections (*1 Fr*)

Fourteen-Day Menu for Men
(1,600 Calories)

Each day's menu provides the following number of servings for each food group: 2 milk (*Mk*), 6 meat (*Mt*), 6 starches (*St*), 4 fruits (*Fr*), 4-plus vegetables (*Vg*), 6 fat (*Ft*).

- To make 1,500 calories: omit 2 fat servings (e.g., use "light" rather than regular margarine, dressings, etc.).

- "Free" foods in the menus are items with negligible calories, so you may eat them freely.

- After completing two weeks, return to Day 1 menu.

- In the menus, tbsp. = tablespoon, tsp. = teaspoon, c. = cup, oz. = ounce

DAY 1

Breakfast

½ c. calcium-fortified orange juice or 1 fresh orange (*1 Fr*)

2 slices whole wheat toast or 1 bagel (*2 St*) with 2 tsp. sugar-free jam/jelly (*Free*) and ½ tsp. peanut butter or 1 tsp. tub margarine (*1 Ft*)

1 c. fat-free milk or yogurt (*1 Mk*)

Lunch

tuna sandwich:

2 slices whole wheat bread (*2 St*)

½ c. water-packed tuna (*2 Mt*) mixed with 1 tbsp. light mayonnaise (*1 Ft*) and ¼ c. apple, celery, and pickle (*Free*)

lettuce and tomato slices (*Free*)

1 large apple (*2 Fr*)

1 c. fat-free milk (*1 Mk*)

Dinner

4 oz. skinless chicken breast (*4 Mt*)

1 small red (new) potato (*1 St*) with butter-flavor spray (*Free*)

½ c. carrots, steamed (*1 Vg*)

½ c. green beans, steamed (*1 Vg*)

2 tsp. margarine for vegetables (*2 Ft*)

1 c. green salad (*Free*) with 1 sliced tomato (*1 Vg*) and 2 tbsp. light dressing (*1 Ft*)

½ c. fresh pineapple chunks (*1 Fr*)

Snack

3 c. microwave light popcorn (*1 St, 1 Ft*)

DAY 2

Breakfast

1 c. cubed or ¼ cantaloupe (*1 Fr*)

1 whole wheat English muffin (*2 St*) with 2 tsp. apple butter (*Free*) and 1 tbsp. peanut butter or 1 tsp. tub margarine (*1 Ft*)

1 c. fat-free milk (*1 Mk*)

Lunch

1 small whole wheat bagel or 2 bread (*2 St*) with 2 oz. low-fat cheese (*2 Mt*)

1 raw carrot, in sticks (*1 Vg*)

1 large pear (*2 Fr*)

1 c. fat-free, sugar-free yogurt, flavored or plain (*1 Mk*)

Dinner

4 oz. broiled fish with lemon (*4 Mt*) with 2 tsp. melted margarine (*2 Ft*)

½ c. corn, steamed (*1 St*)

½ c. Brussels sprouts, steamed (*1 Vg*)

2 tsp. (2 tbsp. light) margarine (*2 Ft*)

1 c. romaine lettuce salad (*Free*) with 1 sliced tomato (*1 Vg*) and 1 tbsp. French or 2 tbsp. light dressing (*1 Ft*)

½ c. fresh fruit salad (*1 Fr*)

Snack

5 whole wheat low-fat Triscuit crackers (*1 St*)

DAY 3

Breakfast

½ banana (*1 Fr*)

½ c. bran flakes or Kashi cereal (*1 St*)

1 tbsp. chopped almonds (*1 Ft*)

1 c. fat-free milk (*1 Mk*)

Lunch

turkey sandwich:

2 slices whole wheat bread (*2 St*)

2 oz. turkey (*2 Mt*)

1 tbsp. light mayonnaise (*1 Ft*)

lettuce, tomato slices (*Free*)

1 large apple (*2 Fr*)

1 c. fat-free milk (*1 Mk*)

Dinner

4 oz. lean beef tenderloin (*4 Mt*)

1 c. brown rice (*2 St*) cooked in broth (*Free*)

½ c. zucchini (*1 Vg*) and ½ c. yellow squash (*1 Vg*) stir-fried in 2 tsp. olive oil (*2 Ft*)

1 spinach salad (*Free*) with 1 small tomato (*1 Vg*), 1 tbsp. walnuts (*1 Ft*) and 2 tbsp. light dressing (*2 Ft*)

1 orange, in sections (*1 Fr*)

Snack

3 graham cracker squares (*1 St*)

DAY 4

Breakfast

2 grapefruit halves (*2 Fr*)

1 small whole wheat bagel (*2 St*) with 1½ tbsp. light cream cheese (*1 Ft*)

1 c. fat-free milk (*1 Mk*)

Lunch

1 small red (new) potato (*1 St*) topped with ½ c. low-fat cottage cheese (*2 Mt*)

1 large romaine lettuce salad (*Free*) with 2 tbsp. dressing (*2 Ft*)

½ c. asparagus, sautéed (*1 Vg*) in 1 tsp. olive oil (*1 Ft*) and lemon juice

1 c. strawberries (*1 Fr*)

Dinner

Spaghetti:

3 oz. 90% lean ground beef, cooked and drained (*3 Mt*), ½ c. meatless spaghetti sauce (*1 St*), over 1 c. spaghetti (*2 St*), 3 tbsp. Parmesan cheese (*1 Mt*)

4 c. raw spinach (½ c. steamed) (*1 Vg*) and ½ c. mushrooms and onions (*1 Vg*), sautéed in 2 tsp. olive oil (*2 Ft*)

½ c. carrots, steamed (*1 Vg*)

1 c. melon, cubed (*1 Fr*)

Snack

8 oz. fat-free, sugar-free lemon yogurt (*1 Mk*)

DAY 5

Breakfast

1 orange or ½ c. blueberries (*1 Fr*)

1 c. oatmeal (*2 St*)

1 tbsp. chopped nuts (*1 Ft*)

1 c. fat-free milk (*1 Mk*)

Lunch

pita turkey sandwich:

1 whole wheat pita pocket (*2 St*)

3 oz. turkey (*2 Mt*)

1 oz. (2 slices) low-fat cheese (*1 Mk*)

lettuce, tomato slices (*Free*)

1 tbsp. light mayonnaise (*1 Ft*)

1 c. grapes (*1 Fr*)

½ c. V8 or tomato juice (*1 Vg*)

Dinner

3 oz. baked seafood (*3 Mt*)

½ c. mashed potatoes (*1 St*) with 1 tbsp. light margarine (*1 Ft*)

1 c. vegetable mix (*2 Vg*) stir-fried with 1 tsp. olive oil (*1 Ft*)

mixed green salad (*Free*) with 1½ tbsp. Italian dressing (*2 Ft*)

1 c. fruit salad (*2 Fr*)

Snack

2 large flavored rice cakes or 1 c. Cheerios (*1 St*)

DAY 6

Breakfast

1 c. fat-free plain yogurt (*1 Mk*) topped with 1 banana (*2 Fr*) and ⅔ c. Kashi Go Lean Crunch (*2 St*) and 1 tbsp. chopped walnuts (*1 Ft*)

Lunch

chef salad:

2 c. mixed salad greens (*Free*) with ½ c. raw broccoli and ½ cup raw cauliflower (*1 Vg*), 1 sliced tomato (*1 Vg*), 3 oz. turkey or ham (*3 Mt*), 1 oz. low-fat cheese (*1 Mt*)

3 to 4 tbsp. light dressing (*2 Ft*)

1 c. vegetable soup or 4 Rye-Krisps (*1 St*)

1 fresh peach (*1 Fr*)

Dinner

2 slices of a medium cheese pizza, thin crust (*2 Mt, 2 St, 2 Ft*)

1 c. cucumber, onion, and tomato salad (*1 Vg*) with 1 tbsp. French dressing (*1 Ft*)

1 c. watermelon (*1 Fr*)

Snack

3 graham cracker squares or 5 low-fat Triscuits (*1 St*) or 16 oz. (2 c.) sugar-free, fat-free hot cocoa (*1 Mk*)

DAY 7

Breakfast

½ c. calcium-fortified orange juice or ½ c. blueberries (*1 Fr*)

2 four-inch whole wheat pancakes (*2 St*) topped with 2 tbsp. light syrup (*1 Ft*) and 2 tbsp. light margarine (*2 Ft*)

1 c. fat-free milk (*1 Mk*)

Lunch

4 oz. roasted skinless chicken breast (*4 Mt*)

1 c. brown rice (*2 St*) cooked in chicken broth (*Free*)

½ c. green peas, steamed (*1 St*)

1 c. carrots, steamed (*2 Vg*) with 1 tsp. margarine (*1 Ft*)

½ c. cabbage, shredded (slaw) (*Free*) with 2 tbsp. light dressing (*1 Ft*)

1 c. cubed or ¼ of a cantaloupe (*1 Fr*)

Snack

1 c. fat-free, sugar-free strawberry yogurt (*1 Mk*)

Dinner

taco salad:

½ c. pinto or kidney beans (*1 St, 1 Mt*), 1 oz. (3 tbsp.) grated low-fat cheese (*1 Mt*), 1 sliced tomato (*1 Vg*), 1 c. raw vegetables (green pepper, carrots, red onions, etc.) (*1 Vg*), 1 c. lettuce (*Free*), 1 corn tortilla, toasted and broken into chips (*1 St*), ¼ c. salsa (*Free*)

1 c. fresh pineapple chunks (*2 Fr*)

Snack

1 c. fat-free, sugar-free yogurt (*1 Mk*)

DAY 8

Breakfast

1 fresh orange (*1 Fr*)

1 whole wheat English muffin (*2 St*) topped with ¼ c. 2% milk mozzarella cheese (*1 Mt*)

1 c. fat-free milk (*1 Mk*)

Lunch

fast-food grilled chicken breast sandwich (no mayonnaise) (*2 St, 3 Mt*)

1 large apple or fruit cup (*2 Fr*)

1 c. fat-free milk (*1 Mk*) or occasional 4 oz. fat-free, sugar-free frozen yogurt

Dinner

vegetarian stir-fry:

Heat in skillet in 3 tsp. oil (*3 Ft*): 1½ c. mixed frozen Japanese vegetables (*3 Vg*), ½ c. diced onions and mushrooms (*1 Vg*)

1 c. steamed brown rice (*2 St*)

tossed salad (*Free*) with 2 tbsp. Italian dressing (*3 Ft*)

½ c. fresh pineapple chunks (*1 Fr*) with ½ c. low-fat cottage cheese (*2 Mt*)

1 fortune cookie (*Free*)

Snack

1 wedge/slice low-fat cheese (*1 Mt*)

DAY 9

Breakfast

¼ cantaloupe (*1 Fr*)

1 small cinnamon-raisin bagel (*2 St*) with 1½ tbsp. light cream cheese (*1 Ft*)

8 oz. fat-free, sugar-free vanilla yogurt (*1 Mk*)

Lunch

1 c. lentil or bean soup (*1 St, 1 Vg, 1 Mt*)

1 c. tossed salad (*Free*) with 2 tbsp. ranch dressing (*2 Ft*) and 3 tbsp. Parmesan cheese (*1 Mt*) and 1 tbsp. walnuts (*1 Ft*)

1 whole wheat roll (*1 St*) with 1 tsp. margarine (*1 Ft*)

½ c. fresh fruit salad (*1 Fr*)

Dinner

3 oz. turkey or skinless chicken breast, roasted (*3 Mt*)

½ c. corn, steamed (*1 St*)

1 c. carrots, steamed (*2 Vg*)

1 tbsp. light margarine (*1 Ft*)

4 c. raw spinach (½ c. cooked) (*1 Vg*), sautéed in 1 tsp. olive oil (*1 Ft*)

15-calorie sugar-free popsicle (*Free*)

Snack

half sandwich:

1 slice whole wheat bread (*1 St*), 1 oz. turkey ham (*1 Mt*), mustard, lettuce, tomato (*Free*)

1 c. grapes (*1 Fr*)

1 c. fat-free milk (*1 Mk*)

DAY 10

Breakfast

1 banana (*2 Fr*)

1 c. shredded wheat (*2 St*)

1 tbsp. chopped nuts (*1 Ft*)

1 c. fat-free milk (*1 Mk*)

Lunch

soft tacos:

3 corn tortillas (*3 St*), 3 oz. skinless, cooked chicken (or ½ c. fat-free refried beans) (*3 Mt*) browned in 1 tsp. oil (*1 Ft*), ¼ diced tomato (*Free*), shredded lettuce (*Free*), 3 tbsp. salsa (*Free*)

1 fresh peach (1 Fr)

Dinner

3 oz. red snapper (*3 Mt*) sautéed in 2 tsp. oil (*2 Ft*)

½ c. red (new) potatoes, grilled (*1 St*)

½ c. yellow squash, grilled (*1 Vg*)

½ c. zucchini, grilled (*1 Vg*)

1 c. red bell pepper, grilled (*1 Vg*)

2 tsp. olive oil for vegetables (*2 Ft*)

2 tbsp. balsamic vinegar (*Free*)

1 small fresh tomato, in wedges (*1 Vg*)

Snack

2 c. (16 oz.) fat-free, sugar-free hot cocoa or 8 oz. fat-free, sugar-free lemon yogurt (*1 Mk*)

1 c. grapes (*1 Fr*)

DAY 11

Breakfast

1 c. fresh strawberries (*1 Fr*) and ⅓ c. Kashi Go Lean Crunch (*1 St*) on top of 8 oz. plain, fat-free yogurt (*1 Mk*)

1 slice whole wheat toast (*1 St*) with 1 tsp. margarine or 1½ tbsp. peanut butter (*1 Ft*)

Lunch

tuna sandwich:

> 2 slices whole wheat bread (*2 St*)
>
> ½ c. water-packed tuna (*2 Mt*) mixed with 1 tbsp. light mayonnaise (*1 Ft*) and 3 tbsp. chopped celery, apple, pickle (*Free*)
>
> lettuce, tomato slices (*Free*)

1 fresh large pear or apple (*2 Fr*)

Dinner

low-calorie frozen dinner (up to 300 cal., 10 g fat) (*3 Mt, 1 St, 1 Vg*)

½ c. broccoli, steamed (*1 Vg*), with 1 tbsp. slivered almonds (*1 Ft*) and 1 tsp. margarine (*1 Ft*)

½ c. carrots, steamed (*1 Vg*)

1 c. grapes (*1 Fr*)

Snack

1 c. fat-free milk (*1 Mk*)

½ small (1 oz.) bagel (*1 St*)

1 oz. low-calorie cheese (*1 Mt*)

DAY 12

Breakfast

1 whole grapefruit (*2 Fr*)

2 fat-free Eggo or Kashi waffles (*2 St*) with 2 tbsp. light syrup (*1 Ft*) and 1 tbsp. light margarine (*1 Ft*)

8 oz. fat-free, sugar-free yogurt or 1 c. fat-free milk (*1 Mk*)

Lunch

cheeseburger:

> 1 whole wheat bun (*2 St*)
>
> 3 oz. 90% lean ground beef patty (*3 Mt*)
>
> 1 slice low-fat cheddar cheese (50 cal./oz.) (*1 Mt*)
>
> lettuce, tomato, mustard (*Free*)

1 c. watermelon slices (*1 Fr*)

1 c. fat-free milk (*1 Mk*) or occasional 4 oz. fat-free, sugar-free pudding snack

Dinner

shrimp creole:

> 1 oz. (5 large) boiled shrimp (*1 Mt*) in ½ c. spaghetti sauce (*1 St*), served over 1 c. brown rice (*2 St*), 2 c. vegetable mix (broccoli, cauliflower, carrots, onions, etc.) (*4 Vg*), stir-fried in 2 tsp. oil (*2 Ft*)

tossed salad (*Free*) with 2 tsp. olive oil (*2 Ft*) and 2 tsp. balsamic vinegar (*Free*)

Snack

1 c. cantaloupe (⅓ melon) (*1 Fr*) with ¼ c. low-fat cottage cheese (*1 Mt*)

DAY 13

Breakfast

½ c. calcium-fortified orange juice or 1 fresh orange (*1 Fr*)

1 whole wheat toast (*1 St*) with 1 tbsp. light margarine (*1 Ft*)

1 poached egg (*1 Mt*)

1 c. fat-free milk (*1 Mk*)

Lunch

pasta salad:

> 1 c. cooked pasta (*2 St*), 1 c. steamed vegetables (broccoli, carrots, red bell pepper) (*2 Vg*), 3 to 4 tbsp. light Italian dressing (*2 Ft*), 3 tbsp. grated Parmesan (*1 Mt*)

spinach salad (*Free*) with ½ c. mandarin or orange slices (*1 Fr*) and 2 tbsp. light Catalina dressing (*1 Ft*)

1 c. fat-free milk (*1 Mk*)

Dinner

fajitas:

2 soft whole wheat tortillas (*2 St*), 4 oz. grilled flank steak (*4 Mt*) marinated in 2 tbsp. lime juice (*Free*) and ½ tsp. fajita seasoning (*Free*), ½ c. onion and bell pepper (*1 Vg*) grilled in 1 tsp. oil (*1 Ft*), ½ c. diced tomato (*1 Vg*), ½ c. shredded lettuce (*Free*)

1 c. fresh pineapple chunks (*2 Fr*)

Snack

3 c. microwave light popcorn (*1 St, 1 Ft*)

DAY 14

Breakfast

½ c. fortified grapefruit juice (*1 Fr*)

1 c. strawberries or ½ c. blueberries (*1 Fr*)

2 four-inch whole wheat pancakes (*2 St*) with 2 tbsp. light syrup (*1 Ft*)

1 c. fat-free milk or yogurt (*1 Mk*)

Lunch

3 oz. skinless chicken breast (*3 Mt*) marinated in 3 tbsp. fat-free Italian dressing (*Free*) and baked, grilled, or broiled

½ c. mashed potatoes (*1 St*) with 1 tsp. (or 1 tbsp. light) margarine (*1 Ft*)

½ c. shredded cabbage (*Free*) with 1 tbsp. coleslaw dressing (*1 Ft*)

1 c. yellow squash, steamed (*2 Vg*)

1 c. green beans, steamed (*2 Vg*)

1 tbsp. light margarine for vegetables (*1 Ft*)

1 c. watermelon slices (*1 Fr*)

Dinner

mini-pizzas:

2 English muffin halves (*2 St*) topped with 1 oz. (3 tbsp.) part-skim mozzarella cheese (*1 Mt*)

2 oz. Canadian bacon or smoked turkey (*2 Mt*)

2 tbsp. mushrooms, sliced (*Free*)

2 tbsp. onion, diced (*Free*)

2 tbsp. green pepper, diced (*Free*), ¼ c. pizza or spaghetti sauce (*Free*)

½ c. mixed fresh fruit (*1 Fr*)

Snack

1 c. Cheerios (*1 St*)

1 c. fat-free milk (*1 Mk*)

Supplements

The recommendations we made in Plan B (chapter 12) for common-sense supplementation are also good for Plan C. This goes for sports supplement beverages, which can be an alternative and healthy meal replacement option for Plan C when convenience becomes an issue. You get consolidated calories with a lot of macronutrient impact.

What about diet supplements? They are widely advertised hot sellers. However, there is no single weight-loss supplement on the market that effectively promotes permanent weight loss. The scientific evidence for such products is extremely weak, including for natural appetite suppressants.

Don't fall for the myth that chromium supplements help you lose weight. If chromium is one of the ingredients in your multivitamin, that's fine. But no credible evidence exists to show that this mineral contributes to weight loss, yet it appears in almost every type of weight-loss product. So persistent is this chromium myth that diet supplement manufacturers will not remove it. To do so, they say, is equivalent to product suicide. Consumers have been brainwashed over the years by advertising and insist on it in their multivitamins.

Epilogue

Move Yourself for Life

> We are made wise not by the recollection of our past, but by the responsibility for our future.
>
> —George Bernard Shaw

In our public lectures we half-jokingly refer to the proliferating new order of inactive *Homo sapiens* as *Homo sedentarius*. While we may get a laugh from our audiences, there is nothing funny about the alarming trend of inactivity and the mass scale of sickness, obesity, shortened longevity, and financial cost to society that it brings. If you want a disturbing glimpse of how bad the situation has become in the last few years, and an idea of the horrendous direction we're headed in, get on the Internet and go to the Web site of the Centers for Disease Control and Prevention (www.cdc.gov). Check out the trends for obesity and diabetes. It looks like we are collectively headed for the graveyard. Is this our future?

Some experts have referred to the health implosion here and abroad as "diseases of comfort" and predict they will become the primary cause of death in this and the following century.

In a 2005 issue of the *Journal of Epidemiology and Community Health*, four prominent public health experts on the international scene—Walter Tsou, past president of the American Public Health Association; David Hunter, past chairman of the U.K. Public Health Association; Peter Sainsbury, past president of the Public Health Association of

Australia; and Bernard Choi, a senior research scientist at Canada's Centre for Chronic Disease Prevention and Control—made a dire observation. They pointed out that the world has started to feel the impact of a "global chronic disease epidemic, which is putting pressure on our health care systems. If uncurbed, a new generation of 'diseases of comfort' (such as those chronic diseases caused by obesity and physical inactivity) will become a major public health problem" and "the primary cause of death" in this and the next century.

These diseases of comfort have emerged as the price that we, as creatures of comfort, are increasingly paying for living in a modern society. "It is inevitable that these diseases will become more common and more disabling if human 'progress' and civilization continue toward better (more comfortable) living, without necessarily considering their effects on health," the authors said. "In the USA, a study of national data has shown that only 3 percent of Americans followed all four of the recommended health rules, namely, don't smoke, maintain a normal weight, eat fruit and vegetables, and get some exercise. The effect of following these lifestyle changes is greater than anything else medicine has to offer."

And medicine does offer a lot. The twentieth century saw great strides in medicine. The era of antibiotics, for instance, enabled us to treat once fatal illnesses and contributed to a great leap in longevity. Indeed, life expectancy increased by nearly three decades during a single century. Computer technology brought us significant improvements in our ability to diagnose previously undetectable illnesses, and enhanced our means of caring for patients with conditions we previously could do little for. Advanced surgical techniques, improvements in anesthesia, modern medications, intensive care units, neonatal intensive care units—these are but a few of the miracles available to us today.

But we stand in danger of overwhelming the medical, financial, and even security resources of our nation unless we do our share. If we do not heed the trends, we will amass a collective health debt we cannot pay. And the cost won't be just in health care itself. As our nation becomes increasingly out of shape, where do we hope to find the military personnel of tomorrow to protect us? What about the firefighters and police officers responsible for our communities? The national pool of active, red-blooded individuals seems to be drying up, and as a consequence, so are the folks we need to keep our nation vibrant and healthy.

We are both upbeat doctors who get out a lot, speak to medical and lay audiences, and attend medical conferences. We have our fingers on the pulse of the national heartbeat, so to speak, and we see promising innovation and developments ahead that we hope can help transform *Homo sedentarius* into *Homo activarius*—the active, vibrant, healthy human.

Physical activity research will bring new methods, technologies, and equipment, and new strategies for getting people to make better behavioral choices and stick with them. We'll have metabolic monitors and motion sensors to make tracking progress easier and more accurate than ever. There'll be no more guessing how many calories you burned today or how many you need to burn tomorrow.

We are getting closer also to identifying with precision what type of specific exercise is best for an individual based on genetics and medical condition.

We have a sense that exercise will soon be thought of as part of standard therapy for medical conditions such as heart disease and certain types of cancer. Hopefully, companies and insurance plans will do even more to push physical activity as a cost-saving strategy.

When all is said and done, however, there's nothing really different between what we tell our patients, and what we are telling you, and what Aristotle and Hippocrates told their peers back in ancient times. We can make the recommendations, but it's up to each and every one of you to steer your behavior in a healthy direction. To get up and get active. To eat better. We hope this book has given you some inspiration and practical ideas for accomplishing that.

We know, from the patients we see and from the research we do, that if individuals don't take charge of their lives, then indeed the "diseases of comfort" will surely take down our current generations and those to follow. We also know just how wonderful, remedial, and life-changing physical activity can be—even a low but regular dose of it—and how contagious the changes can be for friends and family who quickly see the difference.

APPENDIX A
RESOURCES

Cooper Aerobics Center
Call (972) 560-2667 or visit the center's Web site at www.cooperaerobics.com for information on medical services, fitness center, and weight loss programs. For information on research and clinical studies, personal trainer certification, fitness specialty courses, and consulting services, contact the Cooper Institute at (972) 341-3200 or on the Internet at www.cooperinstitute.org, or by mail at 12200 Preston Road, Dallas, TX 75230.

Active Living Every Day
The Active Living Every Day program teaches people to initiate, adopt, and maintain physical activity in their individual lifestyle. For more information on this program and where it is given, call (217) 351-5076, ext. 2226, or visit the Internet Web site www.activeliving.info/.

America on the Move
This national organization is dedicated to helping individuals and communities make positive changes to improve health and quality of life. AOM strives to inspire Americans to engage in fun, simple ways to become more active and eat more healthfully. To find out about affiliated groups near you, call (800) 807-0077 or visit AOM's Internet Web site: aom.americaonthemove.org.

President's Council on Physical Fitness and Sports
The council's informative Web site (www.fitness.gov) contains lots of valuable information on physical activity and links to grass roots organizations that sponsor health and fitness programs.

APPENDIX B
SELECTED REFERENCES

Chapter One. A Little Activity Goes a Long Way

Blair SN, Kohl HW III, Gordon NF. Physical activity and health: a lifestyle approach. *Med Exerc Nutr Health*, 1992;1:54–57.

Blair SN, Kohl HW III, Paffenbarger RS Jr, Cooper KH, et al. Physical fitness and all-cause mortality. A prospective study of healthy men and women. *JAMA*, 1989;262(17):2395–401.

Blair SN, Kohl HW III, Paffenbarger RS Jr, et al. Changes in physical fitness and all-cause mortality. A prospective study of healthy and unhealthy men. *JAMA*, 1995;273(14):1093–8.

Booth FW, Chakravarthy MV, Gordon SE, et al. Waging war on physical inactivity: using modern molecular ammunition against an ancient enemy. *J Appl Physiol*, 2002;93:3–30.

Centers for Disease Control and Prevention. Preventing obesity and chronic diseases through good nutrition and physical activity. July 2005 revision. http://apps.nccd.cdc.gov/EmailForm/print_table.asp.

Centers for Disease Control and Prevention. November 2005. Chronic Disease Overview. www.cdc.gov/nccdphp/overview.htm.

Centers for Disease Control and Prevention. Trends in leisure time physical inactivity by age, sex, and race/ethnicity—United States, 1994–2004. *MMWR*, October 7:54(39):991–94.

Church TS, Earnest CP, Skinner JS, et al. Effects of different doses of physical activity on cardiorespiratory fitness among sedentary, overweight, or obese postmenopausal women with elevated blood pressure: a randomized controlled trial. *JAMA*, 2007;297(19):208–91.

Colditz GA. Economic costs of obesity and inactivity. *Med Sci Sports Exerc*, 1999;31(11 Suppl):S663–7.

Duncan JJ, Gordon NF, Scott CB. Women walking for health and fitness. How much is enough? *JAMA*, 1991;266(23):3295-9.

Dunn AL, Marcus BH, Blair SN, et al. Comparison of lifestyle and structured interventions to increase cardiovascular fitness. *JAMA*, 1999;281:327–34.

Fleg JL, Morrell CH, Bos AG, et al. Accelerated longitudinal decline of aerobic capacity in healthy older adults. *Circulation*, 2005;112(5):674–82.

Garrett NA, Brasure M, Schmitz KH, et al. Physical inactivity: direct cost to a health plan. *Am J Prev Med*, 2004;27(4):304–9.

Jakicic JM, Wing RR, Butler BA, et al. Prescribing exercise in multiple short bouts versus one continuous bout: effects of adherence, cardiorespiratory fitness, and weight loss in overweight women. *Int J Obes Relat Metab Disord*, 1995;19(12):893–901.

Mitchell TL, Gibbons LW, Devers SM, et al. Effects of cardiorespiratory fitness on healthcare utilization. *Med Sci Sports Exerc*, 2004;36(12):2088–92.

President's Council on Physical Fitness and Sports. 2002. Cost and consequences of sedentary living: New battleground for an old enemy. *Research Digest*, March Series 3, no. 16:1–8.

Chapter Two. Focus on Fitness, Not Thinness

Atlantis E, Chow CM, Kirby A, et al. Worksite intervention effects on physical health: a randomized controlled trial. *Health Promot Int*, 2006;21(3): 191–200.

Blair SN, Church TS. The fitness, obesity, and health equation. Is physical activity the common denominator? *JAMA*, 2004; 292(10):1232–3.

Church TS, LaMonte MJ, Barlow CE, et al. Cardiorespiratory fitness and body mass index as predictors of cardiovascular disease mortality among men with diabetes. *Arch Intern Med*, 2005;165:2114–120

Flegal KM, Graubard BI, Williamson DF, et al. Excess deaths associated with underweight, overweight, and obesity. *JAMA*, 2005;293(15):1861–7.

Jagust W, Harvey D, Mungas D, et al. Central obesity and the aging brain. *Arch Neurol*, 2005;62(10):1545–8.

Kay SJ, Fiatarone Singh MA. The influence of physical activity on abdominal fat: a systematic review of the literature. *Obes Rev*, 2006:7(2):183–200.

Klein S, Fontana L, Young VL, et al. Absence of an effect of liposuction on insulin action and risk factors for coronary heart disease. *N Engl J Med*, 2004;350(25):2549–57.

Kuk JL, Katzmarzyk PT, Nichaman MZ, et al. Visceral fat is an independent predictor of all-cause mortality in men. *Obesity*, 2006;14(2):336–41.

Nicklas BJ, Cesari M, Penninx BW, et al. Abdominal obesity is an independent risk factor for chronic heart failure in older people. *J Am Geriatr Soc*, 2006; 54(3):413–20.

Otake S, Takeda H, Suzuki Y, et al. Association of visceral fat accumulation and plasma adiponectin with colorectal adenoma: evidence for participation of insulin resistance. *Clin Cancer Res*, 2005;11(10):3642–6.

Schapira DV, Clark RA, Wolff PA, et al. Visceral obesity and breast cancer risk. *Cancer*, 1994;74(2):632–9.

Srdic B, Stokic E, Polzovic A, et al. Abdominal adipose tissue—significance and methods of detection. *Med Pregl*, 2005;58(5–6):258–64.

Yusuf S, Hawken S, Ounpuu S, et al. Obesity and the risk of myocardial infarction in 27, 000 participants from 52 countries: a case-control study. *Lancet*, 2005;366(9497):1640–9.

Wei M, Kampert JB, Barlow CE, et al. Relationship between low cardio-respiratory fitness and mortality in normal-weight, overweight, and obese men. *JAMA*, 1999;282:1547–53.

Chapter Three. The Healing Miracle of Movement

Hardman AE. Honoring Jeremy Morris with the degree of honorary Doctor of Science. Loughborough University, Leicestershire, UK. December 16, 2002. www.lboro.ac.uk/service/publicity/degree_days/degree_2002/winter2002/jeremy_morris.html.

Move to Stop the Metabolic Syndrome

Bertrais S, Beyeme-Ondoua JP, Czernichow S, et al. Sedentary behaviors, physical activity, and metabolic syndrome in middle-aged French subjects. *Obes Res*, 2005;13(5):936–44.

de Ferranti SD, Gauvreau K, Rifai N, et al. Prevalence of the metabolic syndrome in American adolescents: findings from the Third National Health and Nutrition Examination Survey. *Circulation*, 2004;110:2494–7.

Dunstan DW, Salmon J, Owen N, et al. Associations of TV viewing and physical activity with the metabolic syndrome in Australian adults. *Diabetologia*, 2005;48(11):2254–61.

Elabbassi WN, Haddad HA. The epidemic of the metabolic syndrome. *Saudi Med J*, 2005;26(3):373–5.

Farrell SW, Cheng YJ, Blair SN. Prevalence of the metabolic syndrome across cardiorespiratory fitness levels in women. *Obes Res*, 2004; 12(5):824–30.

Finley CE, LaMonte MJ, Waslien CI, et al. Cardiorespiratory fitness, macronutrient intake, and the metabolic syndrome: the Aerobics Center Longitudinal Study. *J Am Diet Assoc*, 2006;106:673–79.

Ford ES, Kohl HW 3rd, Mokdad AH, et al. Sedentary behavior, physical activity, and the metabolic syndrome among U.S. adults. *Obes Res*, 2005;13(3):608–14.

Heart and Stroke Foundation of Canada. 2004. October 25 press release. ww2.heartandstroke.ca.

Jurca RM, LaMonte MJ, Church TS, et al. Associations of muscle strength and aerobic fitness with metabolic syndrome in men. *Med Sci Sports Exerc*, 2004;36(8): 1301–7.

Katzmarzyk PT, Church TS, Blair SN. Cardiorespiratory fitness attenuates the effects of the metabolic syndrome on all-cause and cardiovascular disease mortality in men. *Arch Intern Med*, 2004;164:109–97.

Katzmarzyk PT, Church TS, Janssen I, et al. Metabolic syndrome, obesity, and mortality: impact of cardiorespiratory fitness. *Diabetes Care*, 2005;28(2):391–7.

LaMonte MJ, Barlow CE, Jurca R, et al. Cardiorespiratory fitness is inversely associated with the incidence of metabolic syndrome: a prospective study of men and women. *Circulation*, 2005;112(4):453–5.

Mori Y, Hoshino K, Yokota K, et al. Differences in the pathology of the metabolic syndrome with or without visceral fat accumulation. *Endocrine*, 2006;29(1):149–54.

Resnick HE, Jones K, Ruotolo G, et al. Insulin resistance, the metabolic syndrome, and risk of incident cardiovascular disease in nondiabetic American Indians. The Strong Heart Study. *Diabetes Care*, 2003; 26:861–7.

Shaw JE, Chisholm DJ. Epidemiology and prevention of type 2 diabetes and the metabolic syndrome. *MJA*, 2003;179(7):379–83

Move against Diabetes

Church TS, LaMonte MJ, Barlow CE, et al. Cardiorespiratory fitness and body mass index as predictors of cardiovascular disease mortality among men with diabetes. *Arch Intern Med*, 2005;165:2114–20

Church TS, Cheng YJ, Earnest CP, et al. Exercise capacity and body composition as predictors or mortality among men with diabetes. *Diabetes Care*, 2004;27(1):83–8.

Diabetes Prevention Program Research Group. Reduction in the incidence of type 2 diabetes with lifestyle intervention or metformin. *New Engl J Med*, 2002;346(6):393–403.

LaMonte MJ, Blair SN, Church TS. Physical activity and diabetes prevention. *J Appl Physiol*, 2005;99:1205–13.

McConnaughey, J. CDC issues diabetes warning for children. Associated Press, June 15, 2003.

Wei M, Gibbons L, Mitchell TL, et al. The association between cardiorespiratory fitness and impaired fasting glucose and type 2 diabetes mellitus in men. *Ann Intern Med*, 1999;130(2):89–96.

World Health Organization. 2002. Statistics on diabetes. www.who.int.

Move against Heart Disease

Church TS, Barlow CE, Earnest CP, et al. Associations between cardiorespiratory fitness and C-reactive protein in men. *Arterioscler Thromb Vasc Biol*, 2002; 22:1869–76.

Church TS, Kampert JB, Gibbons LW, et al. Usefulness of cardiorespiratory fitness as a predictor of all-cause and cardiovascular disease mortality in men with systemic hypertension. *Am J Cardiol*, 2001;88:651–6.

Gibbons L, Mitchell TL, Wei M, et al. The maximal exercise test as a predictor of risk for coronary heart disease mortality in asymptomatic men. *Am J Cardiol*, 2000;86(53):53–8.

Jurca R, Church TS, Morss GM, et al. Eight weeks of moderate-intensity exercise training increases heart rate variability in sedentary postmenopausal women. *Am Heart J*, 2004;147(5):e21.

Lee CD, Blair SN. Cardiorespiratory fitness and stroke mortality in men. *Med Sci Sports Exerc*, 2002;34(4):592–5.

Lee CD, Folsom AR, Blair SN. Physical activity and stroke risk: a meta-analysis. *Stroke*, 2003;34(10):2475–81.

Smith SC, Allen J, Blair SN, et al. AHA/ACC guidelines for secondary prevention for patients with coronary and other atherosclerotic vascular disease: 2006 update. *J Am Coll Cardiol*, 2006;47:2130–9.

Whang W, Manson JE, Hu FB, et al. Physical exertion, exercise, and sudden cardiac death in women. *JAMA*, 2006;295(12):1399–403.

Move against Cancer

Batty D, Thune I. Does physical activity prevent cancer? *BMJ*, 2000; 321:1424–25.

Herrero F, San Juan AF, Fleck SJ, et al. Combined aerobic and resistance training in breast cancer survivors: a randomized, controlled pilot trial. *Int J Sports Med*, 2006;27:573–80.

Holmes MD, Chen WY, Feskanich D, et al. Physical activity and survival after breast cancer diagnosis. *JAMA*, 2005;293(20):2479–86.

Jennen C, Uhlenbruck G. Exercise and life-satisfactory-fitness: complementary strategies in the prevention and rehabilitation of illnesses. *Evid Based Complement Alternat Med*, 2004;1(2):157–65.

Kampert JB, Blair SN, Barlow CE, et al. Physical activity, physical fitness, and all-cause and cancer mortality: a prospective study of men and women. *Ann Epidemiol*, 1996;6(5):452–7.

Lee CD, Blair SN. Cardiorespiratory fitness and smoking-related and total cancer mortality in men. *Med Sci Sports Exerc*, 2002;34(5):735–9.

Lee IM. Physical activity and cancer prevention—data from epidemiologic studies. *Med Sci Sports Exerc*, 2003;35(11):1823–7.

Ohira T, Schmitz KH, Ahmed RL, et al. Effects of weight training on quality of life in recent breast cancer survivors: the Weight Training for Breast Cancer Survivors (WTBS) Study. *Cancer*, 2006;106(9):2076–83.

Schnohr P, Gronbaek M, Petersen L, et al. Physical activity in leisure-time and risk of cancer: 14-year follow-up of 28, 000 Danish men and women. *Scand J Public Health*, 2005;33(4):244–9.

Movement against Osteoporosis

Priest E, Church TS. Association of bone mineral density with cardio-respiratory fitness in men. Paper presented at the Society for Epidemiologic Research, 37th annual meeting, Salt Lake City, Utah, 2004.

Move to Beat Depression

Abbott RD, White LR, Ross GW, et al. Walking and dementia in physically capable elderly men. *JAMA*, 2004;22;292(12):1447–53.

Carney RM, Blumenthal JA, Freedland KE, et al. Low heart rate variability and the effect of depression on post-myocardial infarction mortality. *Arch Intern Med*, 2005;165(13):1486–91.

Dunn AL, Trivedi MH, Kampert JB, et al. Exercise treatment for depression. *Am J Prev Med*, 2005;28(1):1–8.

Galper DI, Trivedi MH, Barlow CE, et al. Inverse association between physical inactivity and mental health in men and women. *Med Sci Sports Exerc*, 2006;38:173–8.

Heyn P, Abreu BC, Ottenbacher KJ. The effects of exercise training on elderly persons with cognitive impairment and dementia: a meta-analysis. *Arch Phys Med Rehabil*, 2004;85(10):1694–704.

Landers, DM. The influence of exercise on mental health. www.fitness.gov/mentalhealth.htm.

Larson EB, Wang L, Bowen JD, et al. Exercise is associated with reduced risk for incident dementia among persons 65 years of age and older. *Ann Intern Med*, 2006;144(2):73–81.

Teri L, Gibbons LE, McCurry SM, et al. Exercise plus behavioral management in patients with Alzheimer disease: a randomized controlled trial. *JAMA*, 2003;290(15):2015–22.

Van Praag H, Shubert T, Gage FH, et al. Exercise enhances learning and hippocampal neurogenesis in aged mice. *J Neurosci*, 2005:25(38):8680–5.

Weuve J, Kang JH, Manson JE, et al. Physical activity, including walking, and cognitive function in older women. *JAMA*, 2004;292(12):1454–61.

Move for More Energy

Holbrook AM. Treating insomnia. *Br Med J*, 2004;329(7476):1198–9.

Powell P, Bentall RP, Nye FJ, et al. Randomized controlled trial of patient education to encourage graded exercise in chronic fatigue syndrome. *Br Med J*, 2001;322(7283):387–90.

Move for Better Sleep

Copinschi G. Metabolic and endocrine effects of sleep deprivation. *Essent Psychopharmacol*, 2005;6(6):341–7.

Tworoger SS, Yasui Y, Vitiello MV. Effects of a yearlong moderate-intensity exercise and a stretching intervention on sleep quality in postmenopausal women. *Sleep*, 2003;26(7):830–36.

Move for Better Sex

Bortz WM II, Wallace DH. Physical fitness, aging, and sexuality. *West J Med*, 1999;170:167–9.

Move for Better Digestion and Elimination

Church TS, Kuk JL, Ross R, et al. Association of cardiorespiratory fitness, body mass index, and waist circumference to nonalcoholic fatty liver disease. *Gastroenterology*, 2006;130:2023–30.

Dukas L, Willett WC, Giovannucci EL. 2003. Association between physical activity, fiber intake, and other lifestyle variables and constipation in a study of women. *Am J Gastroenterol*, 2003;98:1790–6.

Everhart JE, Go VL, Johannes RS, et al. A longitudinal survey of self-reported bowel habits in the United States. *Dig Dis Sci*, 1989;34:1153–62.

Leitzmann MF, Giovannucci EL, Rimm EB, et al. The relation of physical activity to risk for symptomatic gallstone disease in men. *Ann Intern Med*, 1998;128(6):417–25.

Levy RL, Linde JA, Feld KA, et al. The association of gastrointestinal symptoms with weight, diet, and exercise in weight-loss program participants. *Clin Gastroenterol Hepatol*, 2005;3(10):992–6.

Lustyk MK, Jarrett ME, Bennett JC, et al. Does a physically active lifestyle improve symptoms in women with irritable bowel syndrome? *Gastroenterol Nurs*, 2001;24(3):129–37.

Misciagna G, Centonze S, Leoci C, et al. Diet, physical activity, and gallstones—a population-based, case-control study in southern Italy. *Am J Clin Nutr*, 1999;69(1):120–6.

Nguyen-Duy TB, Nichaman MZ, Church TS, Blair SN, Ross R. Visceral fat and liver fat are independent predictors of metabolic risk factors in men. *Am J Physiol Endocrinol Metab*, 2003;284(6):E1065–71.

Whitehead WE, Drinkwater D, Cheskin LJ, et al. Constipation in the elderly living at home. Definition, prevalence, and relationship to lifestyle and health status. *J Am Geriatr Soc*, 1989;37:423–9.

Move to Reduce Pain

Keane GP, Saal JA. The sports medicine approach to occupational low back pain. *West J Med*, 1991;154:525–7.

Richards SC, Scott DL. Prescribed exercise in people with fibromyalgia: parallel group randomized controlled trial. *Br Med J*, 2002;325:185–87.

Move for Headache Relief

Jones AY, Dean E, Lo SK. Interrelationships between anxiety, lifestyle self-reports and fitness in a sample of Hong Kong University students. *Stress*, 2002;5(1):65–71.

Neususs K, Neumann B, Steinhoff BJ, et al. Physical activity and fitness in patients with headache disorders. *Int J Sports Med*, 1997;18(8):607–11.

Rasmussen BK. Migraine and tension-type headache in a general population: precipitating factors, female hormones, sleep pattern and relation to lifestyle. *Pain*, 1993;53(1):65–72.

Move to Live Better Longer

Christmas C, Anderson RA. Exercise in older patients: Guidelines for the clinician. *J Am Geriatr Soc*, 2000;48:318–24.

FitzGerald S, Barlow CE, Kampert JB, et al. Muscular fitness and all-cause mortality: prospective observations. *J Physical Activity and Health*; 2004; 1:6–18.

Simons R, Andel R. The effects of resistance training and walking on functional fitness in advanced old age. *J Aging Health*, 2006;18(1):91–105.

Stein R. It's never too late to be healthy, studies show. *Washington Post*, Sept 22, 2004: A01.

Chapter Five. Step Counting and Logging: Your Keys to Success

Armstrong K, Edwards H. The effectiveness of a pram-walking exercise programme in reducing depressive symptomatology for postnatal women. *Int J Nurs Pract*, 2004;10(4):177–94.

Bassett DR, Schneider PL, Huntington GE. Physical activity in an Old Order Amish community. *Med Sci Sports Exerc*, 2004;36(1):79–85.

Bassett DR, Ainsworth BE, Leggett SR, et al. Accuracy of five electronic pedometers for measuring distance walked. *Med Sci Sports Exerc*, 1996; 28(8):1071–7.

Welk GJ, Differding JA, Thompson RW, et al. The utility of the Digi-Walker step counter to assess daily physical activity patterns. *Med Sci Sports Exerc*, 2000;32(9):S481–88.

Epilogue. Move Yourself for Life

Choi BC, Hunter DJ, Tsou W, Sainsbury P. Diseases of comfort: Primary cause of death in the 22nd century. *J Epidemiol Community Health*, 2005; 59(12):1030–4.

INDEX